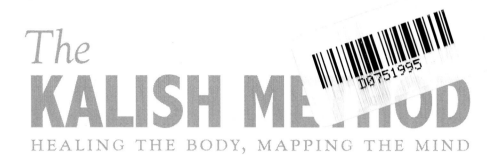

The
KALISH METHOD

HEALING THE BODY, MAPPING THE MIND

DR. DANIEL KALISH

Every effort has been made to ensure that the information contained in this book is complete and accurate. However, neither the author nor the publisher is engaged in rendering advice to the individual reader.

The Kalish Method
Healing the Body, Mapping the Mind

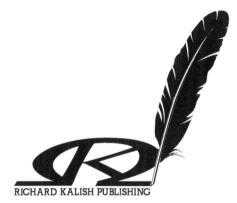

RICHARD KALISH PUBLISHING

Cover Photography: Siddiqi Ray
Cover and Book Design: Carrie Medeiros
Illustrations: Carrie Medeiros
Editor: Matt Olds

Library of Congress Cataloging-in-Publication Data
The Kalish Method: Healing the Body, Mapping the Mind
Daniel Kalish, DC
Library of Congress Control Number: 201290981

To order, visit www.kalishresearch.com

This book is dedicated to my father, Richard Kalish,
researcher and academician by trade,
screenwriter and actor at heart.

ACKNOWLEDGEMENTS

I want to acknowledge all those who made this book a reality. My writing coach Luke Shanahan, who taught me how to bring my writing to a new level. Carrie Medeiros, whose layout work made the book look so good. Matt Olds, for all his fine editing work. Of course, thanks to my patients without whom this book would not be possible. From the work we've done together as a team, you have shown me the remarkable healing power we all hold within ourselves, just waiting to be released.

INTRODUCTION

Do you suffer from fatigue or depression, or are you gaining weight, having digestive problems, or experiencing female hormone imbalances? If so, this book will give you cause for hope. When I began practicing twenty years ago, people suffering from one or more of these debilitating conditions had few places to turn to receive the care they needed to get better. As the years have gone by, my own clinical experience has mirrored what we have all read in the national statistics, with more and more people hit by this set of related disorders—feeling tired, depressed, gaining weight, experiencing heartburn and other digestive problems, and even female hormone issues—collectively, what I call the "Big Five."

I decided I needed to do something about this and so I made it my life's work to educate as many people as possible as to the natural solutions available for these five common problems. Along the way I've learned how to identify those people I can help using the Kalish Method. The Kalish Method employs the modality of functional medicine, so let me tell you what functional medicine is and how this new system of natural healing can help you feel better and find yourself.

Functional medicine uses lab-based natural health programs along with lifestyle changes to reverse all of the Big Five disorders. One of the things I like most about functional medicine is that it's based on laboratory science. At the same time, the rebel in me likes that these functional lab tests differ from conventional lab testing in that they aren't designed to pick up a disease after it occurs, but are instead designed to find health problems early on so they can be effectively reversed with natural therapies, avoiding the unnecessary use of drugs or surgery.

The Kalish Method is not a cure-all; it does not cure cancer, or reverse bone loss or, as you can see from my photo on the cover, baldness. What the Kalish Method does is work incredibly well for the related Big Five conditions. If you suffer from any one of them you've come to the right place.

In the beginning years of my practice I mastered the naturopathic treatments for adrenal hormone imbalances, digestive problems, and detoxification. The first part of this book reflects that heritage of time-tested natural medicine protocols handed down from generation to generation that Dr. Timmins, my first mentor, passed on to me. The second part of my book talks about the new science of the brain. My current mentor, Dr. Hinz, taught me the powerful relationship between toxins in the environment and neurological conditions we see blooming all around us, from autism to ADD. Dr. Hinz has shown me how to heal the brain and how to effectively combat brain disorders, and that there are steps we can take once we understand how to measure these chemicals in the brain. This new area of neuroscience hinges on Dr. Hinz's research findings and represents the next generation of amino acid therapies.

I hope that by the time you are done reading this book you are convinced there is hope out there, and that no matter how sick you feel or how long you've felt that way that there are new tools used by those trained in the Kalish Method that are options to help you start feeling better today.

If you feel like you have lost yourself, or have been taken down by stress and the challenges life has thrown your way, this work can help bring you, the real you, back. No one can escape the effects of chronic stress. The Kalish Method, however, provides a map for you to return, step by step, back to who you really are, healthy, vibrant, content. I can promise you that my clinic is often the treatment of last resort for patients, and that the Kalish Method is where many people go when everything else has failed. My goal for you is to experience what it is like to have perfectly balanced hormones and brain chemicals along with a healthy body; once you have this perfected you can experience the real you. I've heard from hundreds of patients that when their body and brain are finally balanced they feel like a new person, because in a very real way they are.

If you struggle with excess body fat, fatigue, depression, digestive problems, or female hormone issues, you may still believe, and I hope you do, that the real you is inside just waiting to be released. That's how my patients feel and how you're going to feel very soon, if we only give it a try.

This work is not for everyone. You have to admit first, before healing, that much of what we suffer from is self-inflicted: poor diet choices, lack of exercise, and focus on work and career, not on family and relationships. But because we choose these things we can, by choice, go back to a healthier way of being. Functional medicine testing and nutritional programs address one aspect of the problem; the other you must confront on your own, with coaching and support from people like me, so you can regain what you deserve: a healthy body and a healthy mind.

Do you want to experience what that feels like? The Kalish Method can help.

CONTENTS

· ·

WHY DO I FEEL SO CRUMMY, DOC?:
INTRODUCTION TO THE KALISH METHOD

1. FAT, FATIGUED, AND DEPRESSED: THE MODERN EPIDEMIC

How do you feel? If you are like most Americans, chances are you could be feeling better. Given that 62% of Americans are overweight and 21 million people suffer from depression in our country, the odds are you have too much body fat, are fatigued, and/or depressed. If you're reading this book, you've probably already realized traditional medicine can do very little for you.

I have developed a system for correcting what I call the "Big Five" common health problems: weight gain, fatigue, depression, digestive issues, and female hormone imbalances. How did I come up with this list? By treating regular people, folks just like you, day in and day out for 18 years in my natural health clinic. The Big Five include some of the most serious health problems facing us today. And because the standard medical community has done little to address these issues, many people seek my help as an alternative to conventional medicine. Through many years of practice I've developed the Kalish Method to help people suffering from any or all of the Big Five conditions, and you'll learn as we go through this book how it works. You'll come to understand how these problems are related and that they are often the result of a single cause.

Regrettably, these issues have become part and parcel of modern American life, so much so that many people have given up hope that they will ever feel better. I wrote this book to show you that there is indeed hope. Leading health practitioners are employing curative methodologies that were simply unavailable to us as recently as ten years ago. By the time you've finished this book, you'll understand more about the progress that's been made and how you can benefit from these advances. No matter how bad you've been feeling, or how long you've been feeling bad, there are options. You *should* feel better. And with the Kalish Method, *now you can*. Let's look at each of the Big Five in more detail.

Weight Gain

If you struggle with weight gain and have tried various diets only to fail repeatedly in reaching your weight-loss goals, then you most likely suffer from a damaged fat-burning metabolism. If your metabolism is broken, you will store body fat regardless of what or how much you eat. Cravings for sweets or carbs, overeating, skipping meals—all these contribute to a damaged metabolism. Trying to lose weight by following fad diets that restrict calories might allow you to lose weight temporarily, but as soon as you eat normally again, your broken metabolism will put the pounds right back on, and then some.

The more times you have gained and lost weight, the more likely you have damaged your metabolism, and you won't lose weight permanently until you repair it. Many past medical solutions for weight loss such as diet pills and liquid diets make people worse. Fortunately, there is a bright spot in this bleak picture: With the right tests, you can get an accurate picture of your physiological status. Then, with that vital information, you and your health care professional can take steps to correct it. By measuring key hormones such as cortisol, for example, your health professional can figure out how beat up your fat burning system is and what you'll need to do to mend it.

Fatigue

About eight years ago my office manager pulled the charts for every new patient we had seen in the past twelve months and wrote out each person's top three symptoms. Everyone treated that year wrote fatigue as one of their top three concerns. Fatigue most frequently looks like nothing is wrong from a standard medical work up. Doctors often blame it on aging. Heck, most doctors are often exhausted themselves, so to them it seems pretty normal to be tired all the time.

To break this cycle and stop the fatigue a simple test is needed. We measure the energy production systems of the body and, if they are depleted and worn out, boost them back up. Although not routinely used in standard medicine, the test for energy production shows precisely at what times of day your system crashes and what can be done to get things back on track.

Depression

Are you happy? I mean, really happy? Do you wake up and hop out of bed thinking to yourself, I'm going to have a fabulous day! Though you might find it difficult to believe, that's exactly the attitude millions of Americans have. They are really, truly happy. Unfortunately, this kind of happiness is becoming something of a rarity. What is increasingly common is the opposite condition, people waking up feeling as though they'd rather have kept sleeping, held down by feelings of hopelessness and dread. If you are depressed, you likely think of positively joyful people as a little strange, maybe even annoying.

If you're depressed, I want to let you in on some wonderful news: No matter how long you've suffered from depression, you can still become one of those leap-from-your-bed, happy people. I couldn't have made that promise when I first starting practicing. But recently the world of depression treatment has changed: New discoveries now make it possible for your doctor to, in effect, take a kind of "snapshot of your mind" by accurately measuring the neurotransmitter levels in your brain. This crucial new tool means that trained professionals can now pinpoint the imbalances that give

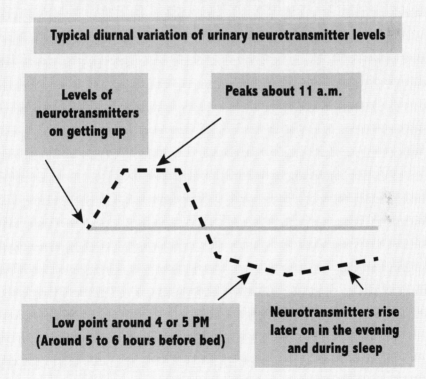

5 TO 6 HOURS BEFORE BED

DIURNAL NEUROTRANSMITTER VARIATION

Typical diurnal variation of urinary neurotransmitter levels

Levels of neurotransmitters on getting up

Peaks about 11 a.m.

Low point around 4 or 5 PM (Around 5 to 6 hours before bed)

Neurotransmitters rise later on in the evening and during sleep

Neurotransmitters are made in a cycle just like hormones. They peak at 11am and drop to their low points around 4pm which is a time many of us feel a drop in energy.

rise to depression and effectively correct them. Without this "snapshot," doctors could only guess at which treatments would be most effective. The tools they were using were simply too blunt to cut the ropes that bound their patients to their chronic depressions. I call the clinical use of these "snapshots" *mind mapping*. I'll discuss mind mapping in detail later.

Digestive Problems

Although embarrassing for sufferers to talk about, heartburn, constipation, diarrhea, gas, and bloating affect most Americans. That means that if you suffer from one or more of these issues, you're not alone. And like many others, you might be so used to these issues that you've come to accept them as normal. A few years ago, I asked a new patient named Beth if she had regular bowel movements. She said yes, they were quite regular. I assumed she meant once a day, so I was shocked when she clarified "regularly once a week." It's not normal to pass gas every day of your life, or to have frequent loose stools. These issues clearly indicate digestive distress, so for your sake (and for the sake of those around you) it makes sense to get these issues remedied.

Female Hormone Imbalances

Most women at some point bump up against symptoms sparked by fluctuations in hormones. Women under age 45 with a ton of stress typically experience PMS-related problems, like cramping, bloating, craving sweets, or premenstrual migraines. In women over age 45, dropping estrogen levels start to create chaos; think hot flashes, night sweats, mood swings, sleep problems, and an unfortunate extra few pounds of body fat around the tummy. Technology developed by my mentor, Dr. William Timmins,

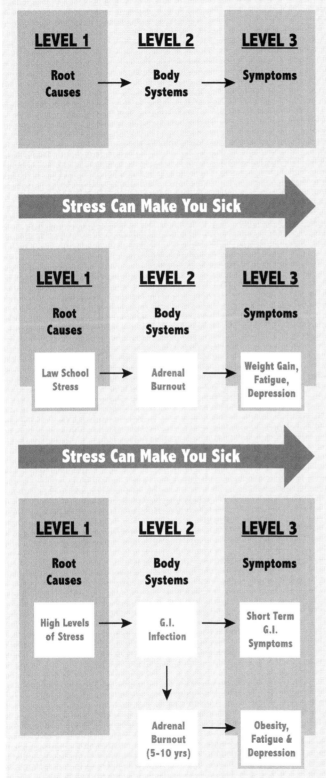

Three levels of functional medicine

Functional medicine focuses on finding the root causes that trigger the three body systems to crash, which in turn is what creates the symptoms we all experience.

High stress levels burn out the adrenal glands and make us prone to weight gain, fatigue, and depression.

Stress and digestive problems combine in many people to create weight gain, fatigue and depression.

now exists to measure female hormone levels throughout the cycle and map out precisely where the problems lie and how to correct them.

What Causes the Big Five Health Issues?

A breakdown in one or more of the *three key body systems* creates the Big Five health issues. These three body systems include the adrenal hormone system, the digestive system, and the liver detox pathways. You don't have to be a doctor to understand how these systems fall apart, yet you might be surprised that a lot of doctors are unaware of how it occurs. I want to help you better understand how your body works and what happens when things go wrong.

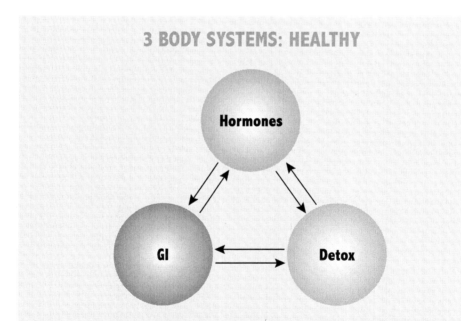

3 BODY SYSTEMS: HEALTHY

When each body system is functioning properly we are healthy and fit, emotionally and physically.

Let's take a look at the three key body systems and see what can cause them to break down:

Adrenal Hormone System (High-stress hormones)

Breakdown from increased cortisol (the main stress hormone) caused by emotional, dietary, and inflammatory problems.

Digestive System (Poor digestion)

Breakdown from food intolerances and the prevalence of "gut bugs."

Liver Detox Pathways (High toxin burden)

Breakdown from exposure to environmental toxins.

Most likely one or more of these body systems has failed in your body and is causing your symptoms. These body systems also interact with one another, so if, for example, your stress hormone cortisol gets out of whack, your digestive health will be impaired. Many people experience this connection between cortisol and digestion, the most common occurrences being the formation of an ulcer or stomach pains during periods of high stress.

High Stress Hormones: The Trigger for Many Health Problems

Do you scream at rude drivers on the freeway, or squeeze your steering wheel with a white-knuckle death grip? Do you vent when your frustrations overboil, or stuff your feelings? Whether expressing or suppressing, high stress equals high cortisol and puts into motion a series of events which culminate in the Big Five. How exactly does this happen? First, the stress response triggers a flood of cortisol, weakening your digestive system lining and making you prone to food reactions and gut bugs. Second, your faltering digestive system then allows high levels of toxins to build up,

As the "mother" of the body, it literally feeds your organs and tissues, from your brain to your adrenal glands, just like a mother feeds her child. Poor digestion leads to poor nutrient absorption, even if you are eating the right foods. The tricky part of this is that, of the people determined through lab tests to have poor digestion, almost half experience no obvious digestive symptoms at all. They have weight gain, fatigue, depression, even female hormone imbalances directly related to poor digestion, but without experiencing heartburn, gas, bloating, and the like. Because digestive symptoms are often masked, discovery of these issues through testing is a critical step.

Digestive problems are caused by two factors: 1) Food reactions, and 2) Pathogens.

1. Food reactions typically involve gluten (wheat), dairy, or soy, which can trigger digestive distress.
2. Pathogens are "bugs" (bad bacterias, yeasts, or parasitic organisms) that invade the gut and create a host of problems.

Blocked Detoxification: Liver detox pathways flounder

If your liver detox pathways are not working well and a buildup of toxins is generated in your body, you will experience an increased risk of developing any one of the Big Five. We store toxins in fat tissue, so more toxins results in the need for more body fat. The body also attempts to buffer the negative impact of some toxins by holding onto fluid, leading to a bloated look and weight gain from fluid retention. Finally, toxins easily enter the brain, damaging brain cells and causing fatigue and depression.

Our liver detox pathways fail for two reasons: 1) the internal generation of toxins which results in a lack of adequate nutrients for running the liver detox pathways properly due to poor digestion and 2) exposure to environmental toxins from food, air, and water. To deal with internally generated toxins, we test and correct the digestive system. External toxins must be avoided as much as possible by taking practical steps like buying organic foods, getting "green" household cleaners, and using water filters. Once you've reduced your exposure to toxins, you can then correct your liver detox pathways using lab-based supplement programs.

If this information has you feeling a bit overwhelmed, know that it is actually simpler than it seems. By understanding the three key body systems, you'll have a good foundation for all the other concepts in this book. When you understand these systems, there's a good chance you will know more about these basic processes than your own physician. Later in the book we will see how these systems interact and how the Kalish Method works synergistically with those interactions. Once you understand these three body systems and can put that information in the context of your personal health history, you'll figure out how you developed your problems in the first place.

2. THE REASONS STANDARD TREATMENTS FAIL

It's a "dark age" of medicine now. TV ads glamorizing drugs and medical procedures are paid for by a pharmaceutical industry desperate for our reliance on medications to solve problems that are really lifestyle driven. (High cholesterol from a bad diet? We have a pill for that!) To make matters worse, doctors today are unable to deal with their patients in-depth to determine the true root of their troubles. Short visits dictated by insurance company payments don't leave time for doctors to focus on teaching people how to de-stress or eat better. But aside from these more easily understood issues, there are other, less obvious but significant reasons why standard treatments fail.

Lack Of Diagnostic Information

It's a tricky balance to achieve, relieving your symptoms while taking the time to assess what the underlying problems may be. It's frustrating to spend time and money hunting for the hidden clues to your actual troubles. It's much easier, and seemingly effective, to just open the medicine cabinet for relief from your immediate symptoms. The problem comes when treatments start before a complete diagnosis is made, and that happens more often than not in conventional medical settings. It is, unfortunately, the easy way out, trying to find a quick fix for whatever ails you. In the worst-case scenario you might benefit from a treatment only to find years later that some underlying cause was not found and that your overall health now suffers because of what was missed earlier.

Overly Focused On Treating Symptoms

In the absence of taking the time to gather accurate diagnostic data from tests, doctors tend to rely on treating symptoms. The problem with symptom suppression-oriented care is that while in the short term it can provide relief, two new problems are set in motion. First, most medications have side-effects which over time start to create their own unique set of difficulties. Second, if there was an underlying cause of the symptoms in the first place, that problem is not being addressed and will typically worsen, eventually causing even more symptoms to pop up. This can play out much like a medical version of the "Whack-A-Mole" arcade game, with desperate attempts at "whacking" new symptoms as they inevitably appear. Over time, people with one underlying cause of poor health can end up with a variety of seemingly disconnected symptoms. Often, each of these symptoms is treated separately and with different medications, and we're off and running in a dangerously misguided new direction.

Ready, Fire, Aim!

Medical treatments for the Big Five can fall short of expectations and tend to follow the "ready, fire, aim" approach, leading off with inadequate information followed by poor treatment decisions. Highly trained in hospital settings, orthodox physicians are never exposed to functional medicine tests or taught to use assessments of the three key body systems to determine proper treatments for the common chronic problems that make up the Big Five. Barriers to learning this information make it challenging for physicians to incorporate these concepts into their practices. The main hurdle for orthodox medicine is that these treatments are based on natural health solutions which do not use medications or surgeries, and so for the most part are seen as outside of conventional medicine's practice.

Conventional Medicine Makes People Worse

The number one rule for health practitioners goes back 2,000 years, "Do No Harm," meaning it is against the rules of medicine to make people worse. The current over-reliance on powerful medications that are not adequately safety tested long-term has created a good deal of harm. Following are five examples of conventional treatments for the Big Five that break the "Do No Harm" decree.

1. Weight Loss Treatments

Most of you struggling with weight loss have a damaged metabolism which blocks your ability to burn body fat. Losing weight while suffering from a broken metabolism forces you into taking extreme and unhealthy measures. The widespread use of the diet pill Fen-Phen stands out as a case in point.

Fenfluramine is a drug that increases levels of serotonin, one of your key neurotransmitters. Phentermine is a psychostimulant drug chemically related to amphetamines, a class of drugs which speeds up your central nervous system with an "adrenaline" rush, hence the street name, "speed." These two drugs (Fen-Phen) were prescribed together to millions of Americans from 1992 to 1997 and were abruptly removed from the market when a study by the Mayo Clinic showed that 30% of Fen-Phen users experienced potentially life-threatening problems with their heart valves.

Not only was the heart damage notable for breaking the "Do No Harm" rule, but the use of amphetamines also caused significant changes to the brain. Of course, while taking these types of drugs your hunger ebbs and you lose weight, but when you come off of these medications there are long-lasting impacts in terms of negative changes to basic brain functions including memory, focus, concentration, and mood. Additionally, when you stop these medications you lose the appetite-suppressing function the drugs provide, resulting in the dieting "rebound" phenomena: You will overeat and put all the weight you lost back on, and then some.

2. Treatments for Fatigue

If you go to a conventional doctor complaining about fatigue, he or she will usually run a battery of lab tests to rule out significant medical problems like anemia, hypothyroidism, even cancer. Once you've been through this process you'll likely be told nothing is wrong. At this juncture, if you accept the diagnosis, you'll usually be reassuringly told, "Don't worry, it's just in your head," or "It's just part of getting older to be tired all the time." Then, if pressed, doctors typically will prescribe an antidepressant that works on your excitatory neurotransmitters, which will initially energize you and boost up your stimulating brain chemicals.

Over time, however, these medications will sap your energy and damage otherwise healthy brain cells, leading to an increased risk of depression, anxiety, and other mood-related problems later on.

3. Treatments for Depression

Depression makes people desperate. There is no other explanation for the popularity of the current conventional treatments which are effective on average 10% of the time and will eventually make you worse. (There is one exception: For those with *major* depression these medications can be helpful, which I will discuss in detail later.) We tragically rely upon a half-baked medical solution for a serious problem that impacts millions of people.

The commonly used antidepressants (such as Zoloft, Prozac, and Wellbutrin) all act through the same basic mechanism which inevitably makes you worse by depleting the very chemicals they are attempting to boost up. These types of drugs block the recycling of brain chemicals back into the cells. In the process of doing this the brain chemicals are left in increasing amounts outside of the cells that protect them, where enzymes then chew them up and destroy them. Over time this accelerated breakdown process

INADEQUATE SEROTONIN AND DOPAMINE LEVELS CAUSE DISEASE

OBESITY

OTHER DISEASES

TYPE II ADULT DIABETES

Decreased Life Expectancy
Diabetes
Heart Disease
Increase in Stroke
Sleep Apnea
Knee Problems
Back Problems
Increased Rehabilitation Time
Increased Rate of Injuries
Increase in Gall Stones
Female Fertility Problems
Gynecologic Irregularities
Gouty Arthritis
High Blood Pressure
Hiatal Hernia
High Cholesterol
Increased Lung Infections
Increase in Gastric Ulcers
Chronic Pain
Fibromyalgia
Myoclonus

Decreased Life Expectancy
Increased Infections
Diabetic Neuropathy
Kidney Failure
Macular Degeneration
Heart Diseases
Foot Ulcers
Vascular Disease
Therapeutic Amputations
Disability
Increase in Stroke
Impotence

HIGH BLOOD PRESSURE AND HIGH CHOLESTEROL

Decreased Life Expectancy
Heart Disease
Stroke
Kidney Failure
Vascular Disease
Ischema

INCREASE CANCER RISK

Increased Colon Cancer
Increased Uterian Cancer
Increased Breast Cancer

Parkinsonism
Obesity
Bullemia
Anorexia
Depression
Anxiety
Panic Attacks
Migraine Headaches
Tension Headaches
Premenstrual
 Syndrome (PMS)
Menopausal Symptoms
Obsessive Compulsive
 Disorder (OCD)
Insomnia
Impulsivity
Obsessionality
Inappropriate Aggression
Inappropriate Anger
Psychotic Illness
Fibromyalgia
Chronic fatigue syndrome
Adrenal fatigue/burnout
Hyperactivity
ADHD/ADD
Hormone dysfunction
Adrenal dysfunction
Dementia
Alzheimer's disease
Traumatic Brain Injury
Phobias
Chronic Pain
Nocturnal Myoclonus
Crohn's Disease
Ulcerative Colitis
Cognitive Deterioration
Functional Deterioration
Increased mortality rate
Organ System Dysfunction
Chronic Stress
Cortisol Dysfunction
Hormone Dysfunction
Restless Leg Syndrome

- Most patients have more than one disease active at any time.

- The incidence of these diseases increases after exposure to drugs that deplete neurotransmitters.

- The key neurotransmitters serotonin and dopamine are found all over the body and imbalances create many symptoms other than ones strictly related to the brain.

lowers your normal levels of brain chemicals, leaving you more depleted each year you take these medications. This rarely mentioned effect isn't even a recent discovery, as it was first uncovered by researchers at M.I.T. in the 1960s. Yes, you read that right—science has known for over 40 years that, over time, antidepressant medications make your brain worse.

4. Heartburn and Stomach Problems

One in twenty Americans now take medication for stomach pain, heartburn, and acid reflux. In the last decade doctors started to treat these types of stomach problems with Prilosec or Zantac, a class of medications called Proton Pump Inhibitors (PPIs). Recent research studies show these drugs make people worse. Yes, they block all but 10% of your stomach acid production and reduce short-term symptoms. However, blocking stomach acid production has its dark side, as it leads to a reduction in nutrient absorption and increased susceptibility to bacterial infections and other gut bugs. Also, when you stop taking the medications there is a nasty rebound effect with a magnification of the original level of stomach pain. Blocking stomach acid relieves one symptom, but causes other moles to pop out of different holes.

These medications alleviate the symptoms so quickly that most people stop wondering why they had heartburn in the first place. The treatment prevents the appropriate diagnosis and allows the underlying problem to continue. Up until the advent of this new class of drugs, doctors would help patients problem-solve this common issue, considering diet, stress, and weight gain. Now you will just be given a drug that makes you worse.

5. Hormone Replacement Therapy and Thelma Amelia Wilson

Hormone replacement therapy was a misguided experiment that went terribly wrong and ended up damaging the lives of tens of thousands of women, leaving behind its legacy of health problems caused by a supposedly helpful treatment. This story shows the harm that can be created by one company advocating the use of a drug treatment that becomes accepted due to good marketing and PR, even when that treatment stands in contrast to all the known science. This started when Dr. Robert Wilson launched his sales campaign for Premarin, a synthetic estrogen, in 1966. Both his book, Feminine Forever, and his sham research foundation were paid for in secret by the pharmaceutical company Wyeth, the manufacturer of Premarin. Based on his falsified research, Premarin eventually climbed to the top-earning position for medications and, in 2001, 45 million prescriptions for hormone replacement therapy (HRT) were written. HRT became the standard, unquestioned, safe treatment for menopausal female hormone complaints of hot flashes, night sweats, low sex drive, mood swings, irritability, and insomnia.

The trouble was that, after 36 years of widespread use, in 2002 The Women's Health Initiative study which included 16,000 participants definitively showed that HRT put women at risk for everything from breast cancer to Alzheimer's to heart disease. Many of these conditions were supposed to be prevented by HRT. It's now accepted in conventional medicine that HRTs' benefits are not worth the risks and that HRT makes you worse. As a sad footnote to the story, Thelma Amelia Wilson, Dr. Wilson's wife, took Premarin and died of estrogen-related breast cancer in 1988.

3. THE KALISH METHOD: A DIFFERENT APPROACH

Development of the Kalish Method

I never intended to create a whole new treatment model. What I wanted to do was help people while working in my small, comfortable, and busy practice in Del Mar, California. Then one day Barbara came to the clinic. A tall and imposing woman from Texas, Barbara took a seat, glared at me, and said these exact words: "I am fat, tired, and depressed, so what are *you* going to *do* about that?"

I had never been confronted by a patient in that way. Barbara challenged me and my authority, but at the same time was direct, honest, and somewhat skeptical yet hopeful because I had already helped so many of her close friends. In my moment of confusion while preparing to respond, I had a flash of realization. Suddenly, my work with patients in the previous years coalesced. Barbara's unexpected directness caused me to finally put all the puzzle pieces together, and in that room on that sunny San Diego day, staring out my window, I came up with my clinical model.

I had treated thousands of patients, and in each case I looked for the exceptions and individual differences. I was treating symptoms while basing my success on being sure people felt better. Barbara's challenge (*What are you going to do about it?*) forced me to see that there was indeed a pattern under all the chaos. I knew I could help her, as I'd already helped six of her close friends with the exact same problems, but suddenly I grasped why. Despite all the variations from patient to patient, I finally saw the obvious: *While the patients and their symptoms and their individual expressions of the problems varied, the underlying problems with the various body systems remained the same.* These similarities were there, hidden from me because my attention was directed towards symptoms and symptom relief.

I now had to throw away focusing on relieving symptoms, which up to that point I'd thought of as my job. Instead of looking at each case as an individual with their own unique problems, now I saw repeating patterns of problems, manifesting as different symptoms. The problems were with the body systems. The symptoms weren't really the problem. Up to this point being happy when patients came back saying their symptoms were gone, I could now only be satisfied when the functions of the key body systems improved.

As I adopted new guiding principles in my pursuit of ignoring symptoms and fixing body systems, I realized there was a three-part process, the one I mentioned earlier that bears repeating:

1. The stress response is the trigger. People start to develop health problems within a year of being under intense emotional stress as their bodies respond to that stress with an increase in cortisol.
2. The high cortisol then causes their digestive systems to fall apart, at least for a little while, sometimes for long periods of time.
3. Eventually toxins build up and their liver detox pathways break down.

All this because Barbara scared the daylights out of me and I had to stammer out a response.

Moving away from symptom-oriented thinking towards a body system model, I finally saw what had been right in front of me all those years of practice. We have three basic body systems that can be thrown off: the adrenals, the digestive system, and our liver detox pathways. Additionally we have the brain and all its regulatory functions. The brain impacts the gut, and the gut impacts the brain. The brain impacts the hormones, and the hormones impact the brain. Toxins impact everything. And to top things

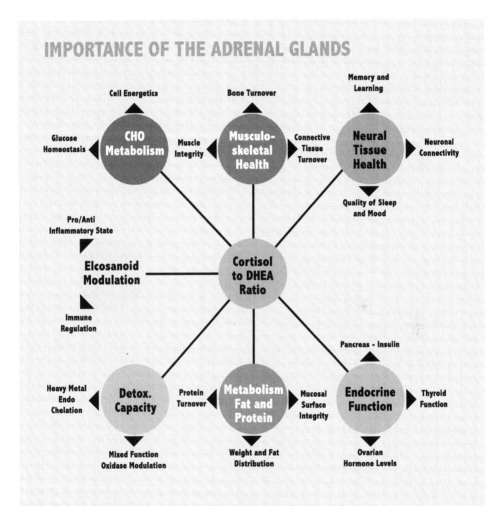

IMPORTANCE OF THE ADRENAL GLANDS

The adrenal glands play a central role in many key body functions.

off, our feelings and thoughts and the emotional events we experience control it all. The complexity of the body was revealed to me in the simple and predictable breakdown patterns of the the three key body systems.

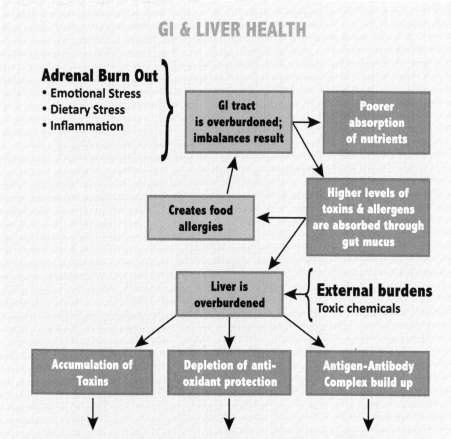

GI & LIVER HEALTH

Adrenal Burn Out
- Emotional Stress
- Dietary Stress
- Inflammation

GI tract is overburdoned; imbalances result

Poorer absorption of nutrients

Creates food allergies

Higher levels of toxins & allergens are absorbed through gut mucus

Liver is overburdened

External burdens
Toxic chemicals

Accumulation of Toxins

Depletion of anti-oxidant protection

Antigen-Antibody Complex build up

WEIGHT GAIN, FATIGUE, DEPRESSION, GI ISSUES, FEMALE HORMONE IMBALANCES

Your body systems are interconnected. When one crashes they are all impacted.

Now, fast forwarding ten years and having applied this model to several thousand new patients and having taught it to hundreds of doctors, I am convinced I have truths to share worthy of your time and consideration.

Adrenal Glands and the Brain

The Kalish Method initially focuses on the first of the three key body systems, the adrenal hormone system, along with the brain (central nervous system and neurotransmitters). Together these form what I call the body's Command System, simply because they serve to maintain overall command of most other body systems. Both the adrenals and the brain can be corrected through a lab-based system of analysis. Now we have a game changer. No longer using symptoms as a reference point for treatment decisions, we use lab tests. No more mole whacking. Using lab-based programs, the results are nothing short of magical.

The Adrenaline Rush

The immediate response to stress is that classic "adrenaline" rush we have all experienced, accompanied by a rush of cortisol to provide the energy we need to act. Cortisol floods your body and stimulates chemicals to rush through your brain, and your adrenal glands and neurotransmitter system go into a state of high alert. But how long can you keep that adrenaline rush going?

Unrelenting stress cranks up these two systems and we end up in go-go-go mode, burning through stress hormones and brain chemicals and depleting that which we require to feel happy, stable, and fit. Living in a state of chronic stress causes the entire Command System to fall apart. The Kalish Method untangles this mess.

Correcting the Command System: Adrenals and Neurotransmitters

Health problems vanish as these two systems come into balance. You will lose weight and have more energy. Mood improves and both digestive problems and female hormone imbalances disappear. It's a miracle every day in my practice, designing programs that heal the adrenal glands and

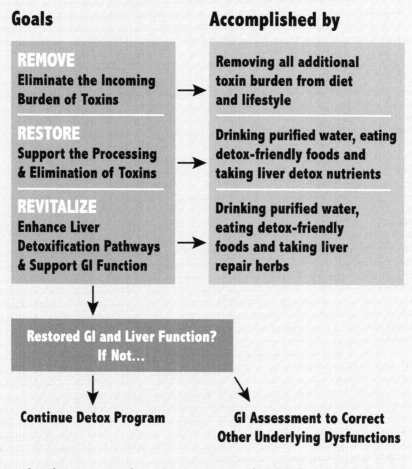

DR. KALISH RENEW PROGRAM GOALS

Goals	Accomplished by
REMOVE Eliminate the Incoming Burden of Toxins	Removing all additional toxin burden from diet and lifestyle
RESTORE Support the Processing & Elimination of Toxins	Drinking purified water, eating detox-friendly foods and taking liver detox nutrients
REVITALIZE Enhance Liver Detoxification Pathways & Support GI Function	Drinking purified water, eating detox-friendly foods and taking liver repair herbs

Restored GI and Liver Function? If Not...

Continue Detox Program

GI Assessment to Correct Other Underlying Dysfunctions

There is a lot you can do to improve your health by eliminating harmful toxins and supporting your detoxification systems.

revitalize the brain. When both the adrenal hormones and brain chemicals are stabilized in concert, your life will change. It's a consistently effective approach. When your car runs out of gas, you add more and it works again. Problem solved. And it's really just as easy with the Kalish Method. In fact, the Kalish Method's very simplicity makes it hard for some to believe. Solving these Big Five problems seems like it should be more complex, but it's not.

My realization that day with Barbara was that her issues with weight gain, fatigue, depression, GI problems, and female hormone imbalances (yes, she had all five) were not all separate and isolated problems. They were five manifestations of one underlying set of problems. And now functional medicine testing will uncover whether you have a primary adrenal hormone imbalance, a primary neurotransmitter imbalance, or a combination of the two, and guide the exact way to the right solution.

Three Stages of Adrenal Exhaustion

Back in the 1950s a famous researcher named Hans Seyle wanted to learn what happens to animals under stress. It turns out that, when stressed, both mice and men react in similar ways. First there is a huge rush of cortisol that fades as we become exhausted. Lots of people actually enjoy this initial feeling of a high-cortisol rush. High cortisol is vital to keep us "up" when we need to be, but when our bodies remain in that go-go-go mode for prolonged periods, eventually things fall apart. As the adrenal glands fail, three stages of adrenal exhaustion can be easily identified by experienced practitioners using a cortisol test. High cortisol, that initial rush stage, is called Stage One. As cortisol drops out and depletes we move into Stage Two, and finally Stage Three is reached when cortisol levels drop to extreme lows and the body begins to shut down. This final stage is characterized by exhaustion, weight gain, and depression. Each of these stages is treated differently. Adrenal hormone imbalances are lifestyle driven, with the three major contributors being emotional stress, dietary stress, and inflammatory stress. The four lifestyle solutions for resolving these adrenal hormone issues are based around diet, exercise, sleep, and stress management, coupled with lab-based nutritional supplement programs. This is how we treat the Big Five.

Neurotransmitter Programs
Within the category of neurotransmitter imbalances, some people suffer from brain chemistry depletion due to stress and lifestyle factors. Others have different issues driving brain chemistry imbalances, which I will describe in a moment.

There are two main neurotransmitters we focus on correcting, serotonin and dopamine. Serotonin is an inhibitory neurotransmitter. Serotonin's functions include the following:
1. Calming you down
2. Relieving anxiety
3. Improving your sleep

Dopamine is an excitatory neurotransmitter. Dopamine's functions include the following:
1. Energizing or "boosting" you up
2. Generating motivation
3. Improving your focus, concentration, and memory

Serotonin and dopamine working together help to control our sense of appetite and cravings for sweets and carbs, and so play a significant role in weight loss programs. Some 95% of the serotonin in the human body is found in the digestive tract, where it controls digestive functions like peristalsis (the gentle contractions of the intestines which facilitate digestion). When abnormal levels of serotonin exist in the gut, people can experience symptoms of irritable bowel syndrome (IBS) or Crohn's disease. And lastly, female hormones and brain chemicals are constantly interacting. Many female hormone imbalances can also be corrected by normalizing serotonin and dopamine.

Three Different Types of Neurotransmitter Problems

If your brain is not fully engaged, you might be suffering from any one of three different types of neurotransmitter imbalances, all of which are treated in similar ways.

1. Deficiency Type: Neurotransmitter levels are low and need to be built back up. Primarily lifestyle and stress driven.

2. Damaged Neuron Bundle Type: Nerve cells have been partially destroyed, requiring greater than expected levels of neurotransmitters to generate normal firing, independent of a person's lifestyle factors. This damage can occur from physical trauma to the brain (traumatic brain injury, TBI), or from chemicals or environmental toxins that destroy brain cells (neurotoxin damage).

3. Genetic Type: Defects in enzyme production result in an inability to make adequate amounts of these chemicals. This issue exists outside the realm of lifestyle factors, as people are born with these genetic issues and have little control over them.

Having Both Adrenal and Brain Problems

Some people suffer from both adrenal- and neurotransmitter-related problems. Indeed, you are entitled to more than one problem at the same time. Some people have lifestyle-generated issues that impact their hormones and brain, and at the same time they may have neuron bundle damage from a series of concussions. These patients demonstrate poor lab findings on both types of testing, and so we then need to hunker down and prepare integrated programs to treat all aspects of the neuroendocrine system.

In the next chapter I will tell how the three key body systems work and how the disruption of these systems can eventually lead to the manifestation of the Big Five. Later on we will cover in detail how the brain plays a role in all this. First we'll look at healing the body, then at healing the mind. By examining the adrenal system, digestive system, and liver detoxification pathways we can typically determine the underlying causes of these all too common health concerns and then develop effective treatment protocols to relieve your symptoms.

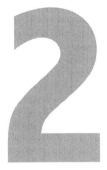

ATTACK OF THE BODY SNATCHERS:

HOW THE MAJOR BODY SYSTEMS ARE DISRUPTED

In Chapter One I talked about the importance of the three key body systems and how the breakdown of these systems results in weight gain, fatigue, depression, digestive problems, and female hormone imbalances—the Big Five. Now it is time to put the pieces together more clearly, and look at how these body systems are disrupted. Once you understand this process, you can then look at your own health history and figure out not only what went wrong, but most importantly how to make things right.

I'd first like to look at each of these three body systems in detail. We'll start with the adrenal hormones, then cover the digestive system, and finally look at the liver detoxification pathways. Once this material is covered you'll see how chronic stress, nutrient deficiency, and toxic overload are the trio of assaults that culminate in the Big Five.

ADRENAL HORMONE SYSTEM

The adrenal hormone system is like the emergency command and control center of your body, or the 911 call center operator. In life or death situations the adrenal hormone cortisol kicks in and tells the other body systems what to do to survive the crisis. When you are under stress, cortisol shuts down fat burning to preserve fuel and gives you a short-term shot of energy called an "adrenaline rush." Cortisol also shuts down the digestive tract and shunts your blood to the muscles so you can fight back or run away. High cortisol inhibits immune system functions because your body gets focused on survival, so repair and healing are luxuries you can't afford. If you stay in this high-alert, high-stress mode for long, cortisol levels crash down, and as they drop you'll develop symptoms, the residual impact of high-stress hormones now being depleted.

When the adrenal glands burn out and cortisol production wanes, you end up storing body fat around the abdominal organs in your belly, your energy level drops and fatigue sets in, and your mood becomes depressed as your cortisol levels are depressed. Eventually some people start to develop ulcers, heartburn, or other digestive problems, and for women the burn out of cortisol burns out the sex hormones, leading to female hormone imbalances. The list of what high cortisol does goes on and on. It destroys the heart and cardiovascular function, and fries the brain, triggering memory loss and cognitive decline. Literally thousands of research studies show that poor cortisol levels translate to long-term degenerative diseases including heart disease, diabetes, and even cancer. In the short term, people with suboptimal cortisol levels suffer from problems that include all of the Big Five.

THREE SOURCES OF ADRENAL DYSFUNCTION

1. Stress Exhausts the Adrenals

Busy people make a lot of cortisol. If you have a deadline at work, you'll make more cortisol to stimulate your brain to help you think clearly. That's fine, but if you work non-stop under constant deadlines for three years without a vacation, your cortisol will burn out. Running late to meet a friend, cortisol floods your blood stream with glucose (sugar), the fuel source you need to hustle up and move faster. If you're late once in a while it's no big deal, but if you are stuck in traffic running late every day, your adrenals will get exhausted. Stress itself isn't harmful, as stress actually motivates us to get things done, but chronic stress is deadly. Moments of stress bracketed by long periods of rest keep us vibrant and engaged and moving forward in life. Chronic, long-lasting stress breaks us down.

The bad situation turns worse if you overdo things and push too hard for too long, as then the high cortisol levels can't turn off. It's like opening a faucet fully and then having the handle break—you just can't stop the flow. Even at night when you should be resting you'll be overly revved up and have trouble sleeping. Adrenal exhaustion means you can no longer turn off the high cortisol, leaving you stuck in fight or flight survival mode. When this goes on year after year you'll start to burn out, exhausting your adrenals. Then the "wired and tired" problems begin. As I've mentioned before, this leads to the Big Five: You'll gain weight and fatigue will set in, and digestive problems and even female hormone symptoms will start to show up. All are absolutely predictable results of adrenal fatigue, as they are just a sign of your body's breakdown. Then, to make a bad situation worse, the longer you have adrenal problems the more likely one of the other primary body systems will be dragged into this downward spiral.

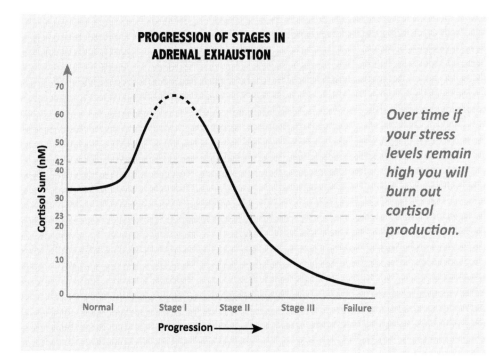

PROGRESSION OF STAGES IN
ADRENAL EXHAUSTION

Over time if your stress levels remain high you will burn out cortisol production.

There's a consistent pattern to all this, and if you have enough problems with cortisol it's just a matter of time until your digestive troubles begin.

2. Nutrient Deficiency from Poor Diet

In one of my favorite movies, The Road to Wellville, with two of my favorite actors, John Cusack and Anthony Hopkins, Hopkins plays the central character Dr. Kellogg, now known for his breakfast cereal idea, who really was one of the original doctors that emphasized the importance of good digestion to overall health. In real life Kellogg had the same zest and passion I aspire to, although in the film he's portrayed as being a little crazy. The human body hasn't changed much in the last 100 years and, like Kellogg, I've also discovered that if you have any of what I call the Big Five problems then most likely your digestion isn't working very well, and will need addressing as a central component of your getting better. The good news is there are only two issues to worry about: Either (1) you're reacting to eating the wrong foods, or (2) there could be some type of infection in your digestive tract.

The digestive problems I'm talking about include heartburn, bloating, gas, constipation, and diarrhea. To figure out where these problems come from we just investigate foods and infections. In terms of food reactions there is a simple way to figure out what's going on. I've had the best results simply by getting patients to eliminate gluten, dairy, and soy for 60 days. At the end of the 60 days they can reintroduce whatever foods they have been missing and have pancakes for breakfast, pizza for lunch, and pasta for dinner for three days and see what happens. You'll find all the details on this in the diet information in the last part of the book.

Digestive tract infections, or "gut bugs," are the second common cause of digestive problems. These require lab testing to figure out. I think you'd be surprised and maybe a little horrified how easy it is to pick up these infections. About 80% of the people I test have some form of infection. You could have parasites, bacteria, or yeast (*Candida*) overgrowth. What's confusing is that you don't have to go somewhere exotic to pick up a gut bug, as parasites are lurking at your local salad bar or public restroom, or on the tongue of that dog that just licked your hand. If you need to, you can put the book down, go wash your hands well in hot soapy water, and come back for the next section in a minute!

Both food reactions and "gut bugs" cause the same type of tissue damage and inflammation in the digestive tract and block nutrient absorption. This lack of nutrients then goes on to create problems in the other body systems. Without enough nutrients, our fat-burning metabolism gets damaged, we can't make enough energy inside our cells, hormone levels drop, and we eventually get fat, fatigued, and depressed. And although this might seem a little repetitive at this point, here we are again, right back at the Big Five.

3. Toxins

Just to review, there are three ways the adrenal glands can go haywire: too much stress, bad digestion, or what we'll discuss now, toxins. Here's a true toxin story for you: Last year I went to a family get-together in Cleveland, Ohio and was forced to leave my very well thought out, pure, and non-toxic lifestyle in California. My house has air purifiers and water filters, I have farm-fresh food delivered, I only use non-toxic cleaners, and I even buy organic clothes! Well, on the first day of my trip to Cleveland I was assaulted with nasty vinyl chloride chemicals off-gassing from the new-model rental car, followed by highly chlorinated water in the hotel shower, and I soon found myself in a full-on, California-boy health crisis. I actually felt pretty sick most of that trip, but it made me appreciate the benefits of getting these toxins out of our lives. Most of the time we just don't think much about the levels of toxins we are exposed to every day because we don't notice them. My trip to Cleveland highlighted how far I'd come in cleaning up my own home and work environment and how avoiding toxins can make a difference in how we feel day to day.

It's impossible to avoid toxins altogether, and so another part of keeping the liver detox pathways working well is to tune them up regularly with supplements that get the liver to dump out any chemicals, or heavy metals that have accumulated in your body's fat tissue. In a perfect world this would happen with a good diet, but these days there are too many environmental toxins for your body to handle on its own and you'll almost certainly need extra support from nutritional supplements. In the Kalish Method of functional medicine, I measure patients' liver detox pathways and then fix them using sulfur-containing amino acids, antioxidants, and vitamins.

Neurotoxins: The Worst Offenders

While we are discussing toxins, I would like to point out neurotoxins, the most persistent and dangerous of all toxin types. I've been aware of the dangers of toxins for 30 years but thought of them more as an abstract problem, like global warming, not as something that could directly impact my life. Then, about three years ago while analyzing lab results at work, I had the sudden realization that the levels of neurotoxins in my patients' labs exactly matched the level of brain cell damage on the neurotransmitter tests they performed. I'd been looking at this data measuring toxin levels and brain cell damage levels for years when finally the connection became obvious, and it suddenly all made sense. The more lead, mercury, or arsenic in your system, the more likely some of your brain cells will be destroyed. In an unfortunate design flaw, you don't have a "dead brain cell warning light" on your forehead. You can't feel this happening. The only warning sign you may have would be the effect these toxins exert on your liver detox pathways. And you can probably guess the rest: Just as with the other body systems, as the liver detox pathways sputter and fail, the Big Five start to appear.

The moral of this story is that any one of the three key body systems can crash (adrenals, digestion, or liver detox pathways), and often it's a combination of all three. One primary system like the adrenals can mess up another primary system, like your digestive system, and it can work the other way also, as the digestive system can contribute to an adrenal problem. These interactions between the body systems are complex, and eventually out of this chaotic mix of dysfunction, symptoms pop up that we notice. If you are experiencing any of the Big Five, the first consideration is to unravel which body systems have been most affected, and then see if you can put together for yourself to just what extent stress, poor nutrition, and/or toxins have contributed to your current problems. Once you have this way of looking at things figured out, whatever health problems you have should start to make perfect sense and you'll be ready to address the next phase, which we'll discuss in Chapter Three, Healing the Body.

GLUTEN QUESTIONNAIRE

Gluten intolerance has been found to be most common among people of Irish, English, Scottish, Scandinavian, and Eastern European descent. Often times it is assumed that gluten intolerance is a food allergy, but it is not. It is actually an autoimmune process, which affects an alarming percentage of the population. The most significant symptoms are weight gain, fatigue and depression.

The following test is a diagnostic tool to help you to understand the symptoms and signs that are likely to go along with gluten intolerance.

TEST INTERPRETATION GUIDE (combine both sections)	
Number of "Yes" Responses	Potential for Gluten Intolerance
4 or less	Not likely
5 – 8	Suspected
9 or more	Very likely

DO ANY OF THE FOLLOWING APPLY TO YOU?		
Yes	No	
		Weight gain
		Unexplained fatigue
		Difficulty relaxing, feel tense frequently
		Unexplained digestive problems
		Female hormone imbalances, (PMS, menopausal symptoms)
		Muscle or joint pain or stiffness of unknown cause
		Migraine like headaches

DO ANY OF THE FOLLOWING APPLY TO YOU? (CONT.)

Yes	No	
		Food allergies/sensitivities
		Difficulty digesting dairy products
		Tendency to over consume alcohol
		Overly sensitive to physical and emotional pain, cry easily
		Cravings for sweets, bread, carbohydrates
		Tendency to overeat sweets, bread, carbohydrates
		Abdominal pain or cramping
		Abdominal bloating or distention
		Intestinal gas
		"Love" specific foods
		Eat when upset, eat to relax
		Constipation or diarrhea of no known cause
		Unexplained skin problems/rashes
		Difficulty gaining weight

HAVE YOU SUFFERED FROM ANY OF THE FOLLOWING CONDITIONS?

Yes	No	
		Allergies
		Depression
		Anorexia
		Bulimia
		Rosacea
		Diabetes
		Osteoporosis/bone loss
		Iron deficiency/anemia
		Chronic fatigue
		Crohn's disease
		Ulcerative colitis

HAVE YOU SUFFERED FROM ANY OF THE FOLLOWING CONDITIONS? (CONT.)

Yes	No	
		Candida
		Hypoglycemia
		Lactose intolerance
		Alcoholism

A BRIEF EXPLANATION OF GLUTEN INTOLERANCE

As stated above, gluten intolerance is an autoimmune process, and not a food allergy. It is most common among people of Irish, English, Scottish, Scandinavian, and Eastern European descent. The most common symptoms include, but are not limited to: **weight gain, fatigue,** and **depression**.

A person with gluten intolerance cannot digest the protein portion of many commonly eaten grains. When this protein is ingested it combines with the enzyme transglutaminase to form an immune complex that deposits on the lining of the intestines. The body recognizes this as a foreign substance, and begins an immune reaction to the complex. Immune cells come into the area and release a series of toxins to try to "kill" this unidentified immune complex. These toxins from the immune system cause inflammation in the digestive system and damage the lining tissue. This is what causes unexplained digestive symptoms like bloating, diarrhea, constipation, gas, and cramping. The toxins are also responsible for feelings of fatigue and malaise after a meal containing these foods.

The walls of the digestive tract are lined with immune cells that form a protective barrier called Secretory IgA. This lining protects against infectious agents such as bacteria, parasites, and fungus. If a person with gluten intolerance continues to eat gluten, in time the constant inflammation and irritation in the digestive tract wears away the Secretory IgA. This depletion of immune cells makes a person's body very susceptible to infectious agents it would normally be able to fight off. The inflammation also begins to damage the small intestine. This affects the person's ability to absorb the nutrients they need. You quite literally are what you eat, and if your body isn't able to properly absorb your food, you will suffer a myriad of symptoms.

The number one symptom associated with malabsorption resulting from gluten intolerance is a combination of fatigue and weight gain. If you are not properly absorbing your food you will not be getting enough of the nutrients from the food you eat. This will leave you constantly hungry and endlessly tired. Without proper absorption of nutrients, mineral and vitamin deficiencies can develop. Muscle cramping is a common symptom that can arise. The lack of magnesium impairs muscle contraction. Magnesium deficiency has also been linked to cardiovascular disease. An inability to absorb calcium can lead to osteoporosis. Mineral deficiency can also create feelings of restlessness and an inability to relax. It can also make sleep difficult and create insomnia. If you cannot absorb your B vitamins you will develop weakness, fatigue, and malaise. If you cannot absorb fats then you cannot control inflammation and since most hormones are made from cholesterol, you will not have the building blocks to synthesize hormones. This among other things can create hormone imbalances, interfering with your ability to handle stress and maintain a balanced emotional state. This also contributes to weight gain in a substantial way. Your hormones have a large effect on your metabolism and your ability to process fats and carbohydrates. Imbalance in insulin will eventually lead to diabetes.

There is also a phenomenon that causes people to crave things that they are allergic to. There are many theories as to why this happens and the exact mechanism is not yet fully understood. But this is the reason why many people crave carbohydrates or become "addicted" to them much the way an alcoholic becomes addicted to alcohol.

There are cells lining the intestinal tract that create enzymes to digest food. They too are damaged in this process. If the body cannot secrete the enzyme lactase, lactose can no longer be digested and the person becomes intolerant to dairy. They may also lose their ability to digest protein, which can lead to a deficiency in amino acids. Amino acids are the building blocks for neurotransmitters, one of which is serotonin. Low levels of serotonin have been medically linked to problems with depression and insomnia.

Eventually the digestive tract develops gaps in areas of constant inflammation. This condition is referred to as leaky gut syndrome. When this occurs, these immune complexes from the gluten reaction—other food particles, parasites, bacteria, viruses, fungi, and any other invaders—can exit the GI tract and enter the blood stream. This increases the body's susceptibility to illness. It is also the origin of many food allergies. Food is meant to be fully digested, broken down, and filtered through the liver before it ever enters the blood stream. As undigested food particles slip through the gaps into the blood stream, the body's immune system sees them as foreign invaders and creates immune cells to them. The next time you eat these foods the body remembers them as a potentially threatening invader and creates a reaction to them resulting in a food allergy.

How to Take Further Action

These are possible reactions that *can* occur over time with a person who is gluten intolerant. Not all people will react in an extreme way, but if you do have intolerance to gluten it is very important that you identify it and avoid all products containing gluten.

If you scored 5 or higher on the questionnaire, I recommend you eliminate all gluten-containing foods from your diet for a minimum of two months. At the end of the two months you will notice significant relief (if not elimination) of your symptoms if you are in fact gluten intolerant. If you identify yourself as gluten intolerant you will need to remain gluten-free for the rest of your life to avoid the unwanted and harmful effects of gluten.

Gluten-free means avoiding all foods containing gluten, including wheat, rye, spelt, bulgur, semolina, couscous, and durum flour. Gluten can be hidden, so read labels carefully. Be wary of modified food starch, dextrin, flavorings and extracts, hydrolyzed vegetable protein, imitation seafood, and creamed or thickened products such as soups, stews, and sauces.

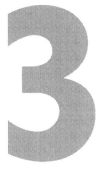

HEALING THE BODY:
THE KALISH PROTOCOL, PHASE ONE

Where to start? That's the question I hear most from the doctors in my training program. With so much information and so many different techniques, doctors and patients alike can become overwhelmed. The Kalish Method presents a simple clinical model rooted in functional medicine. It is the result of decades of clinical expertise, both my own and those of the doctors that trained me. Entirely based on lab testing for analysis, the Kalish Method uses the synergistic coupling of cutting-edge science with natural health treatments which have been used for thousands of years.

Your health problems have come about due to a failure of one or more of your three key body systems. My job as a functional medicine practitioner begins with performing lab tests for each body system to fix what is needed using non-drug, non-surgical methods, including nutritional supplements, herbs, and the like. To make this approach work even better, the Kalish Method incorporates four key lifestyle changes: diet, exercise, stress management, and sleep. This system works incredibly well for the right people with the right problems.

How do you know if you and the Kalish Method are a good match? If you are motivated to make changes in your lifestyle, like eating healthier or reducing stress through yoga classes, this method is right for you. I find that people who are a bit skeptical and cynical do well as long as they are willing to try a few new things and see if they work. In other words, you don't have to be a "believer," you just need to be willing to try. And you don't have to overhaul your entire existence by buying Birkenstocks and going to the Green Festival. Just a few changes, one by one, are enough. The conditions you might have that respond the most consistently and favorably are the Big Five: weight gain, fatigue, depression, digestive issues, and female hormone imbalances, though you can treat a wide variety of problems with these exact same methods.

Let's take a look at how this actually works in the clinic setting and what the treatment experience and results can look like from your perspective.

THE KALISH METHOD IN PRACTICE

Charlene was a young woman I met early in my practice who had the misfortune of being injured in five separate car accidents throughout her life. The one injury that wouldn't clear up, however, was a minor injury from her least severe crash. It just didn't make sense. One day, desperately trying to piece her puzzle together, I happened to ask her about events occurring in her life around the time of that one particular accident. She said it had been during her divorce, and a flash went off in my head. Was it the emotional stress she was going through that had impacted her recovery, more so even than the physical impact she experienced in the accident? As my curiosity about this question grew, I started asking every patient two pretty basic questions, which you can ask yourself right now: "When did your health problems first start?" and "What was going on in your life around that time?" Think loss or grief, like Charlene's divorce, the death of a loved one, the end of an intimate relationship, or maybe an extended financial crisis.

In the years that followed, as I spoke with a wide range of people coming into the clinic, I discovered that although each person's story was compelling and unique, they had one underlying commonality which is likely true for yours, as well. Your original health problems have a 95% chance of happening within a year or so of your being under emotional stress. It will usually be grief or loss, sometimes financial pressures or over-working, and even good stress can be the culprit, like having kids or getting a major promotion. The confusing part of this is that your original health problems are probably not what are bothering you the most today. Take Scott, for example, a tech company CEO who suffered from depression for over a year. We finally traced the origins of his problem to six years earlier when he started his company and began working 80 plus hours a week. Although he'd only felt depressed for a year, the fatigue underlying his depression had actually started with his increased work schedule and mental stress years earlier.

The Kalish Method suggests that you are most vulnerable to developing one or more of the Big Five health problems during a period of extreme (or excessive) stress in your life. As your adrenal glands burn out, digestive problems result, and eventually a buildup of toxins occurs in your body. The key point is that this can be easily reversed when you understand where your problems came from in the first place. My whole goal in writing this book is to explain how this works so you'll have a better understanding about your body and your problems than most conventional physicians ever could. Then you can make your own decisions about how to best proceed.

Addressing the Body Systems

So that's a nice news flash, that stress makes us sick. As Barbara would say, "So what are you going to do about it?" The way we get into a health crisis actually shows us the way out, as we fix the problems in the order in which they occurred. Picture yourself riding a bike on a sunny day when suddenly the chain slips, breaking the gear shifter. If the bike mechanic decides to fix the bike by replacing the gear shifter and ignores the slipping chain, you intuitively will know he's missing something. WHY did the chain slip? What CAUSED it to slip? The broken shifter is merely the result (or the symptom) of what caused the chain to slip in the first place. So the first step is to fix the problem with the chain, and then address the damage it caused. We don't skip a step. The Kalish Method clinical model implies that 95% of the time stress is the "Big Bang" that gives birth to a universe of health issues, so we must correct your adrenal hormone problems first.

Treating Stress Hormones

To fix your problems in the order they occurred, the first step is to test and correct the adrenal hormones cortisol and DHEA. The most accurate way to do this is to measure your cortisol four times in a 24-hour period, using a series of saliva samples which map out your individual circadian rhythm, or 24-hour biological clock. This specific mapping of your unique circadian rhythm reveals a wealth of information about your body, including energy levels and shifts in mood. It will even show your fat burning metabolism in black and white on the lab report, telling the practitioner what issues to address.

How did you get into trouble with cortisol in the first place? When you are stressed your cortisol levels shoot up, and if you remain stressed for an extended period of time, such as a year or two, eventually your cortisol levels "stick" and remain high every day, all day long. It's like constantly flooring the gas pedal as you drive, even when you are at a stop light. This is not a maintainable scenario. After a couple years of pumping out such high levels of cortisol, your adrenal glands start to burn out and, like a car

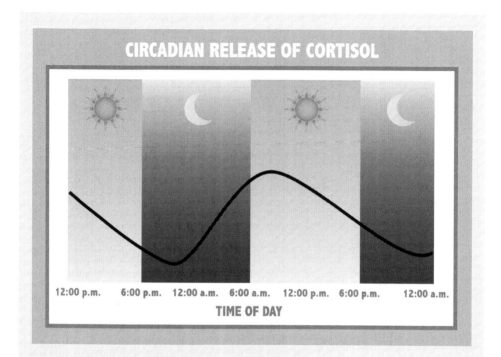

CIRCADIAN RELEASE OF CORTISOL

| 12:00 p.m. | 6:00 p.m. | 12:00 a.m. | 6:00 a.m. | 12:00 p.m. | 6:00 p.m. | 12:00 a.m. |

TIME OF DAY

Hormones, like cortisol, have their production synced up with our exposure to light and dark. Cortisol peaks when we wake up in the early morning and drops throughout the day.

runs out of gas, your cortisol levels plummet. As your cortisol drops lower and lower, your body response of weight gain, fatigue, and depression is set in motion.

Based on your test results, a trained practitioner can determine exactly what stage of adrenal exhaustion you are in. In the very beginning of the burnout process you'll be at Stage One. You'll have extremely high cortisol levels throughout the day and still be in go-go-go mode, like Sheila, a 38-year-old mom with three young kids who had a total cortisol of 180 units per day when the optimum range is 36-42! If you're like this we need to slow things down to restore normal function. Sheila's main complaint was a late-afternoon crash. She was so busy in the mornings that she skipped breakfast completely (although she managed to feed her kids), just grabbing some coffee and heading out for the day. Sometimes Sheila's stage is referred to as "wired and tired" because she'd experience ups and downs throughout the day. If you are at Stage One too, you'll start to crave caffeine in the mornings and sugar in the afternoons. You will probably feel physically ok for the most part, and since you can still make plenty of cortisol, many of the more severe symptoms won't show up yet. Oftentimes if you are in this stage you will think you can get by on five hours of sleep a night, skip breakfast, not take breaks, and still be all right. Many people in Stage One are in a full-time job or go full-time to school, or both, or are raising kids, with no downtime, always on. Or, as the saying goes, "Burning the candle at both ends."

After several years at Stage One, you will drop into Stage Two. Marc, a computer programmer, was extremely sedentary. After a long day at work he'd go home, flip open his laptop, and spend his free-time on the computer. He started to gain weight and lost any interest in exercise. If you are like Marc and have progressed into Stage Two, you'll now have low cortisol and just be entering into a place where one or more of the Big Five symptoms becomes a problem. You'll gain some weight, maybe five or ten pounds. One day you'll want an extra cup of coffee to get through the day, and you won't have the energy to go out after work like you used to. Marc was tired all the time, and sleeping in on the weekends no longer worked to recharge him. Marc's mood was somewhat depressed, and he was just beginning to experience his first digestive symptom, heartburn.

As time marches on, if you continue to let things go, you'll reach Stage Three, like Karen, a 48-year-old executive who runs her own medium-sized company. Her cortisol levels plummeted to 12 units (remember Sheila's cortisol level was 180!), one third of the optimum amount. As CEO she was responsible for everything: new accounts, managing her team, making sure her products got out on time. Karen was up every morning by 5 a.m., exercising, plus working nights and weekends. I had to get her to promise to stop texting and emailing after 6 p.m. and to put the phone down on the weekends. Though Karen was active and had a good diet, her work and family pressures completely exhausted her. She felt depleted, far from her sparkly, high-energy, normal self. If you are at Stage Three, like Karen, with very low cortisol, a one-week vacation won't refresh you; you'll come home tired and dreading returning to work. Exercise will soon become a chore and you'll be too tired to get much done, other than the essentials. With very low cortisol you might just chalk up how you are feeling to aging, but eventually, like Karen, you'll realize something is wrong.

How can you solve these problems? How can you figure out exactly what stage you are in and what you need to do to get better? After 18 years of practice, I have created a straightforward system for you to follow:
1. You take a lab test and have the results explained to you by a practitioner trained in The Kalish Method
2. You start a supplement program based on the lab results which will correct your body's imbalances
3. You make some, but not too many, lifestyle changes

If you are like Sheila and have high cortisol, specific supplements will bring it down. If you have low cortisol, like Karen, different nutrients and herbs will bring it back up. It will seem miraculous as your cortisol returns to normal and your symptoms start to clear up. You'll become healthy again, full of energy and ready to reengage fully in life.

As expected from the three key body systems concept, more advanced stages of adrenal exhaustion imply the development of digestive problems as well. If that's the case, then a complete solution requires one additional test for the digestive system to get that sorted out along with the adrenal program. If caught early enough in the process, then just fixing the first body system, the adrenals, will be enough to get your recovery back on track.

Testing and Correcting the Digestive System

If you are unfortunate enough to have digestive tract problems like gas, bloating, diarrhea, or constipation, believe me when I say that I know they can be an uncomfortable topic to discuss. I had serious digestive problems for 14 years and tried to hide them as much as possible. Eventually with just one lab test, one dietary change, and one treatment program my symptoms cleared up in a few months for good. This experience inspired me to learn how to effectively treat this condition and help folks like you.

The good news is that only two digestive tract problems show up consistently, and when these two problems are taken care of properly, digestive symptoms quickly disappear. These two problems are undesirable food reactions, and having some form of gut bug. To solve the food-related issues, we eliminate gluten, dairy, and soy from your diet for several months. The details on the recommended diet changes are in the back of the book. For gut bugs, we test and figure out exactly which ones you have, and then design a program using antibiotics or herbs to eliminate them and get your digestive system working properly again. Taken together, these two solutions end up generating fantastic results and become a major source of lasting relief from these uncomfortable problems.

Correcting the Liver Detox Pathways

The third and final step is to test and correct the liver detox pathways. Again going back to our Three Key Body System model which explains the progression or development of health problems, if you have let things slide and both your adrenal system and digestive system have collapsed, then most likely your liver detox pathways are overwhelmed. If we've caught things early in the process we can skip this step and just work on the first one or two body systems alone and that will be enough.

Your liver functions like a filter, cleaning up the junk circulating in your blood stream, pulling out chemicals and toxins that could harm your brain and flushing them out of your body. Just like with the adrenals and digestive system there's a test for the liver detox pathways. Based on a urine sample you can do at home, the liver detox pathways test shows exactly what went wrong and what specific nutrients you will need to boost your liver's functioning so it can flush out toxins efficiently.

Treatments

Since I have taught doctors this work and watched it applied in many practice settings, from large medical centers to small, boutique chiropractic or acupuncture clinics, I better understand what The Kalish Method can do. The Kalish Method of functional medicine works consistently for weight loss, fatigue, depression, digestive problems, and female hormone imbalances. Of course it doesn't stop with just those problems. There is also a long history of using functional medicine with far more complex diseases including autoimmune illnesses, addiction recovery, neurological conditions, migraines, thyroid problems, and chronic inflammatory issues. Many chronic conditions benefit from The Kalish Method as a starting point for treatment.

If you step back for a moment and take a big picture view of this, you'll see that the Big Five conditions share a few important characteristics: (1) They are incredibly common, showing up nowadays in the majority of Americans. (2) They are not handled well by orthodox medicine and can even be made worse by traditional treatments. (3) Finally, as you will see in the next section, they respond remarkably well to The Kalish Method. You may be interested to know that my clinical model is so effective it is now in use by medical doctors, chiropractors, naturopaths, and nutritionists. Hundreds of practitioners who have taken my training program apply it in clinics worldwide.

THE CASE STUDIES

Sally

When Sally first came to me she was experiencing fatigue to the point she couldn't exercise, which, being a life-long runner, was a great disappointment. At age 53, she was also more than 20 pounds overweight and was at the end of her rope emotionally: anxious, depressed, and moody. Like a lot of people I work with, she couldn't make many of the lifestyle changes happen initially because she was so exhausted and burned-out she couldn't get around to doing the things she knew were good for her. Eating sweets and living on caffeine every day, she was getting worse and worse, continually putting on extra pounds and getting more desperate for solutions.

After explaining to Sally how breakdowns in the three key body systems generate health problems, she recognized that most of her health issues started a few years after her divorce. The toll of the divorce on her was profound: She lost her will to exercise, her weight ballooned, she became depressed, and these variables compounded until she woke up one day barely recognizing herself and wondering how she got to be in such bad shape.

Sally, like most people I work with, knew she was in trouble and had to regain her health, but she needed a boost and a clear direction to move in. I tested her adrenal glands and hormones, and her digestive system and liver detox pathways. We found her cortisol levels to be quite low, which was depressing her energy levels and making her body store fat. Her low cortisol was also lowering her mood and creating an exhaustion-dominated depression. She wasn't sad, she just didn't have the motivation to get out and do anything.

Her digestive panel showed the presence of a yeast overgrowth called *Candida albicans*, but fortunately her liver detox pathways were fine. We started her on a cortisol-boosting program using very small dosages of pregnenolone, DHEA, and licorice root extract. She also took a multivitamin to provide the vitamins, minerals, and other nutrients—including magnesium, vitamin C, and pantothenic acid (B5)—needed to improve her adrenal hormones.

Within two weeks of beginning the adrenal program, Sally started to pick back up and feel her normal energy return. By the end of the first month she was tentatively exercising and getting back to some of her old routines. In month two we stepped up the program and started to clear out the Candida in her gut. Her sugar cravings stopped and she started to lose weight. Over the course of the first three months of the program Sally lost 10 pounds without dieting, and around that time she decided her energy had sufficiently returned that she could start working out and running. The remaining ten pounds of body fat came off during this phase.

By the end of the sixth month her life was back on track. The short-term dependency on the supplements was fading, and she'd replaced that with her old exercise habits which now gave her the zip and energy she'd been missing. Having taken 20 pounds off her frame, she was fitting in her clothes again and feeling good about herself. Sally, like hundreds of other women her age, was able to restore her adrenal hormones and get back on track with a pinch of lab testing combined with a dash of will power.

Jerry

Jerry is a 42-year-old business owner with three children and a very busy life. He had a long history of digestive problems that had previously been somewhat ambiguously diagnosed as Irritable Bowel Syndrome, or IBS. His company was successful, and he was stressed not due to negative events, but because he simply had so many balls in the air at one time. Running sales meetings and directing trips to soccer games, he didn't get any significant time to himself. The digestive problems had come and gone since his early twenties, and when he was in college he figured out that there were some foods he just couldn't tolerate. He realized that if he stuck to a certain diet he could get by all right, but still with some discomfort. He avoided spicy food and dairy and did ok. Once he hit his 30s, and even with his dietary restrictions in place, he noticed his digestive problems were getting worse. Constant gas and bloating became a problem and he alternated between periods of diarrhea and constipation.

Eventually, when he hit 40, he went to see a gastroenterologist who diagnosed him as having IBS and suggested he follow a high-carb, low-fat diet. Eating tons of pasta and bread for a few weeks made Jerry worse, so he stopped following the doctor's advice and went back to his own devices, avoiding spicy foods and milk products. The IBS kept getting worse and by the time Jerry came in to see me he was having to rush to the toilet occasionally and was worried that his digestive problems were going to interfere with his work.

I ran an adrenal stress test, a digestive panel, and a liver detox profile. Jerry turned out to have moderate problems in all three body systems, so we started off treating his Stage Three adrenal burnout with supplements and immediately focused on his digestive system. The digestive testing showed he had two different microscopic intestinal parasites. He took antibiotics followed by an aggressive herbal program, and after some initial challenges Jerry's digestive problems started to gradually clear up. After six weeks on the program he noticed some normal days without any GI upset at all, and by the three-month mark his IBS symptoms were under control. The only time he would flare up was if he ate the wrong thing, and at this point he had complete control over the IBS if he avoided gluten and dairy products.

Cheating on the diet always brought the symptoms back. After a few months of flare-ups, Jerry decided to go 100% gluten- and dairy-free, and he hasn't had any problems with his digestion since.

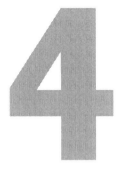

THE PHARMACEUTICAL DART GAME
CURRENT TREATMENTS FOR DEPRESSION, ANXIETY, MOOD DISORDERS, AND ADDICTION

It's getting to the point where I'm no fun anymore
I am sorry

Sometimes it hurts so much I must cry out loud
I am lonely

- Stephen Stills from the song "Judy Blue Eyes"

What would be the worst possible disease you could imagine, the most caustic and destructive condition, something that literally rips apart the fabric of your mind and body, with damaging ripple effects engulfing children, entire families, friends, and communities? My answer to that question is *depression*. Have you ever known someone to survive a heart attack only to end up committing suicide? Of course not. People who survive heart attacks often come back with a goal to lead long lives, and undertake an immediate major reorganization of their priorities, starting with daily exercise and a better diet. My father, Richard Kalish, a social psychologist who spent 30 years studying our attitudes towards death and dying, found that the near-death experience can be a revitalizing event. But what about a disease like depression, where the actual damage isn't to your heart, but the workings of your brain? Motivation and life meaning are stripped from you by the actual process of the disease itself. There's no, "Wow, I really appreciate the little things around me now that I'm depressed." The brain damage itself yanks love for the world around us, love for others, and even love for ourselves away.

When depression deepens, people sometimes turn to suicide. There is no silver lining in a broken brain. Meanwhile, the number of people becoming depressed increases each year, and 15% of adults, or one in six, will experience a major depression. Why are our brains more vulnerable now than 100 years ago? Everyone knows that exercise and diet reduce your risk of heart disease, obesity, or diabetes, but what can you do to protect yourself from depression? This chapter will review the conventional medical treatments available for depression.

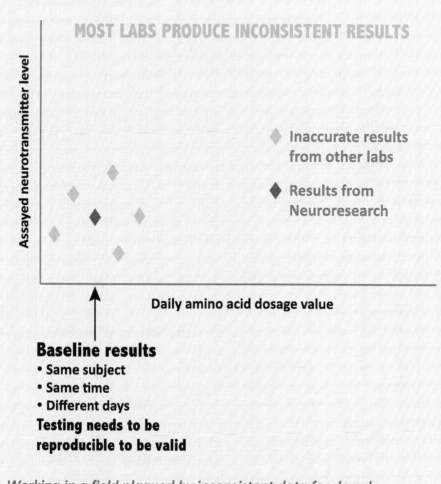

MOST LABS PRODUCE INCONSISTENT RESULTS

Assayed neurotransmitter level

◆ Inaccurate results from other labs

◆ Results from Neuroresearch

Daily amino acid dosage value

Baseline results
• Same subject
• Same time
• Different days
Testing needs to be reproducible to be valid

Working in a field plagued by inconsistent data for decades, Dr. Hinz's lab Neuroresearch has uncovered the secret to measuring neurotransmitter levels. We now have a consistent, reproducible model for mapping brain chemicals, which is key to successful treatment.

Right now most physicians believe that low levels of chemical messengers in the brain, called neurotransmitters, are the culprits in this epidemic. You may have heard or read about some of them, with scientific names like serotonin, dopamine, epinephrine, and norepinephrine. Almost all of the current treatments for depression now in widespread use attempt to manipulate the levels of these chemicals in the brain.

What is Depression?

What does the word depression mean to you? As a medical term it's confusing, because unlike "heart attack," which contains a specific meaning to all of us, we each use the word "depression" in a variety of contexts. For example, you might be "depressed" because you had a car repair that's going to cost $2,000. You'd be bummed for a few days or maybe a week and then get through it. My father's research looked at people's reactions to the death of a loved one. This event might put them into a "depressed" place for several months or a year, but eventually they would pull out of it and move on with life, no longer "depressed" every day. These situational depressions, triggered by life events, are normal and inevitable. When we talk about "major depression," however, it's a whole different world.

The official medical definition of depression says you must have three symptoms: depressed mood, anhedonia (lack of interest in pleasure), and reduced energy. Depression is also rated on a scale consisting of mild, moderate, and major depression. Dana, a previous patient, suffered from major depression. She reached a point where she couldn't take care of herself anymore; she couldn't prepare food or shower, she wore the same clothes every day, and she didn't leave her bedroom. When she made a suicide attempt her family finally had to have her hospitalized. That's major depression.

Less severe symptoms occur with mild and moderate depression. If you have mild depression you might be tired all the time, collapse on the couch every evening after work, and not have the energy to go out and do things other than what's required to keep your life going, like grocery shopping. You've probably stopped exercising and let your diet fall apart, eating sugar and carbs in excessive amounts. You've probably put on weight. Moderate depression lies between the two, not severe enough to consider psychiatric hospitalization, but enough to prevent your having a functional life. This type of depression is referred to in medicine as unipolar depression (*uni* meaning one), because it's one consistent downward spiral with no "up" phase.

Thanks to the current overuse of stimulant psychotropic medications (like Adderall and Ritalin) used to treat Attention Deficit Disorder (ADD), there is now an increased chance of developing a different type of depression called bipolar depression (*bi* meaning two). The two "poles" of bipolar refer to the cycling characteristics of this disease. Bipolar people cycle up and down. There is a manic, or "overly energized," period followed by a harrowing crash.

Causes of Depression

Why would your brain stop working normally? Though your brain is the seat of consciousness, it is still a physical object, an organ inside your head. While the brain has deep mystery to it, it follows the same basic degenerative pattern as other physical objects we are all familiar with. Think of the cars you've owned throughout your life, and the ways in which they deteriorated. It's not so different with your brain. For instance, cars may breakdown from:

1. Wear and tear (lack of regular maintenance or general overuse)

2. Crashes (severe enough impact can cause significant damage)

3. Just being a "Lemon" (remember the Ford Pinto and all the recalls?)

Your brain follows the same basic rules. Broken brains are caused by:

1. Necessary brain chemicals not getting made due to a lack of nutrients required for their synthesis. This can be the result of a bad diet, or from overuse—the more you worry, and get anxious and stressed out, the faster your brain wears out.

2. Trauma, or brain cell damage resulting from either physical injury or nerve toxins.

3. Gene expression, or people who are born with problematic brains stemming from bad genes.

Causes of Depression: The Three Types

There is no clear understanding of how depression occurs. Just as people with normal cholesterol die from heart attacks, serotonin isn't the only variable with depression. Depression can have many different causes. To clarify this, I've developed several categories of causes of depression, including:

1. **Deficiency Type** - a necessary component to normal brain function is missing, such as a nutrient or hormone.

2. **Damage Type** - physical or chemical damage has occurred to the brain. The trauma could be from physical impact or from neurotoxic compounds, such as lead or mercury.

3. **Genetic Type** - people can be born with a genetic predisposition to develop some type of brain problem.

1. DEFICIENCY TYPE

Lack of Exercise

In a 1999 study, researchers at Duke University determined that exercising 30 minutes five times a week reduces depression, confirming a long-held belief. What was truly surprising about the findings was that exercise actually worked better in alleviating depression than a leading antidepressant, Zoloft. Many additional research studies have confirmed that inactivity fosters depression. It's more helpful to get off the couch and walk or jog around the block for 30 minutes a day than it is to drive to a pharmacy and fill an antidepressant prescription.

Low Vitamin D Levels

Do you get a bit down when it's cloudy or rainy out, or when winter comes on and the days get shorter and shorter? It's not your imagination, as lack of sunshine can cause depression. When sunshine strikes our skin, a chemical reaction occurs, forming vitamin D in our bodies. Vitamin D, which is technically a hormone, perks up your mood and your immune system. Lack of exposure to the sun results in low levels of vitamin D, making you feel blue.

Lack of Fatty Acids, Low Vitamin B6

In the documentary film *Supersize Me*, Morgan Turlock vows to only eat at McDonalds for 30 days, breakfast, lunch, and dinner. By the end of the month this previously vibrant, healthy man is reduced to a fat, depressed, sugar-addicted monster. This film provides a clear demonstration of how nutrients from the foods we eat impact how we feel. A lack of healthy fats or a lack of vitamin B6 can set depression in motion. Ideally, you will get the nutrients that stave off depression from omega-3 fish oils. Vitamin B6 is found in meat and fish.

Low Hormones

Barbara, at age 47, had every possible hormone running low: thyroid, estrogen, progesterone, and even testosterone. As one of these alone could cause depression, it was unsurprising that Barbara felt depleted. If you are a woman over age 40 suffering from depression, a drop in hormones could be a contributing factor. The complicated thing about hormones is that for women it's normal for estrogen and progesterone to drop around peri-menopause, and if there is a small problem already lurking in the background, this age-related drop of hormones can create serious problems quite suddenly.

Medication-Induced Deficiencies

Given the level of product-safety obsession we have in America, from automobile floor mat safety recalls to warnings of dangerous toys every Christmas, you would think someone would be pointing out the clear and present danger of the antidepressant medications that are so casually prescribed. We hand them out to kids and adults like they were M&M candies.

To better understand the dangers of the antidepressant medications, I want you to compare serotonin, the brain's feel-good chemical, with a batch of chocolate chip cookies. Let's say that, in your kitchen at home, the batch of chocolate chip cookies is kept in a tin. Members of your family help themselves to one or two cookies, and then get on with their day. But then one day you bake the cookies and leave them out on a plate. Now, people see the cookies sitting there and, unable to resist the temptation, gobble them up much faster than they normally would. This is similar to what can happen with serotonin during depression. Under normal, non-medicated circumstances, your brain makes a batch of serotonin in cells called pre-synaptic neurons. These cells then squirt the serotonin into the synaptic cleft, or synapse, where it hits up against the next brain cell in line (called the post-synaptic neuron). That cell then fires off a signal. Now that its job of communicating messages is done, the serotonin gets sucked back up into the cell that made it. This recycling process is called "reuptake." The gates that open to usher the serotonin back into the cell are called "reuptake ports."

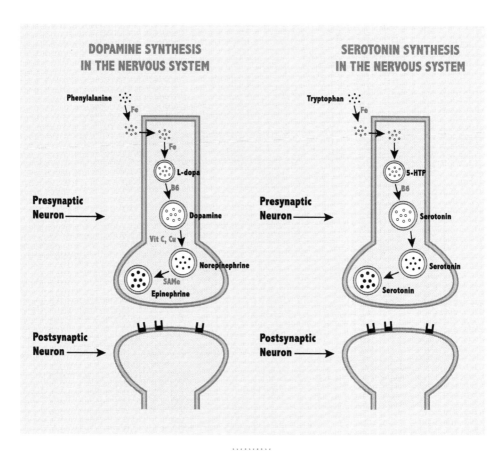

The reason your body pulls the serotonin back into the cell is the same reason your mom put her homemade cookies in a cookie tin: to keep them from being gobbled up. If serotonin is left outside the cell, it will be destroyed at a rapid rate by enzymes whose job is to "clean up" the area around your cells. When the serotonin is pulled back into the cell, it's protected from the enzyme-breakdown process. This detailed bit of knowledge becomes extremely important later in this book.

The implications of this biochemical process are profound but not often talked about. This means anyone who has ever taken any SSRI-based antidepressant has experienced an overall depletion of serotonin. Every year these medications are taken, while the level of serotonin outside the cells goes up from the drug action, the total amount of serotonin in your brain drops because, as I mentioned, the serotonin is degraded by enzymes at a more rapid rate when it is outside the cell. Eventually this shell game collapses and the levels of serotonin in the entire system get so low that the drugs stop working entirely, leaving the brain in far worse shape than it was before. As previously mentioned, this basic mechanism of drug-related depletion of neurotransmitters was first discovered at M.I.T., the U.S.'s top research university, in the 1960s. So why, after 40 plus years, hasn't this finding that antidepressants deplete the very chemicals needed for optimal brain function made the news? This mostly unknown side of the story needs to be understood by anyone considering taking an SSRI.

2. DAMAGE TYPE

Damage Type refers to the actual destruction of nerve cells, rather than something depleting brain chemicals. If you experience a Deficiency

Type problem, we can boost chemical levels and your system will work again. With a Damage Type problem we need to address the cause of the damage, as a broken brain can't just bounce back on its own. It takes more work and perseverance to successfully treat this condition than a Deficiency Type problem.

Post-Synaptic Neuron Receptor Changes

If you remember back to the pre- and post-synaptic neuron concept, the second cell in line, the post-synaptic neuron, operates like a light switch. When you flick the switch, electricity flows, and the light bulb illuminates. Similarly, when serotonin strikes the second cell, it "triggers" that cell's switch, and the cell fires off an electrical signal. If you take an antidepressant medication, you end up with more serotonin in the space between cells, which causes that post-synaptic neuron to grow more receptors. The problem is that as serotonin drops more and more from the drug-induced depletion, the receptors stay in place. This means at the end of the process you have less serotonin but more post-synaptic cell receptor sites, a further recipe for brain disasters. Steve Hyman, former head of the NIMH and Provost of Harvard University, has written entire scientific papers on this one subject: long-term changes to brain cell receptors created by the use of antidepressants. These drugs can change your brain forever, even after you stop taking them.

Traumatic Brain Injury (TBI)

A soldier is riding in an armored Humvee in Iraq when suddenly a roadside bomb explodes, releasing massive waves of energy. A five-year-old falls off the playground monkey bars and hits her head on the concrete below. Concussions come in all sizes. TBI (Traumatic Brain Injury) refers to damage to the brain from physical injury. The forces of the impact cause bleeding and bruising in the brain as it is bounced around inside the head, striking up against the hard, inflexible bones of the skull. While the extent of the damage varies widely depending on your history of injuries, this type of trauma destroys neurons, and once damaged they can't conduct electrical signals properly.

Neurotoxins

For some reason, many nerve poisons, or neurotoxins, seem to have three letter acronyms: DDT, PVC, PCB. All of us that grew up in industrialized countries have some level of exposure to these chemicals. DDT was sprayed on crops for decades until banned because of its dangers to the nervous system. More recently, PVCs, used to soften plastics, were found to cause neurological damage and were banned from use in children's toys. Many of you may have the old-style metal or amalgam fillings which are now known to gradually release the potent neurotoxin mercury. Today it is impossible to eliminate your exposure to environmental neurotoxins.

So why is this of such importance? Problems begin when one of these tiny neurotoxic molecules penetrates your brain and contacts one of your nerve cells. Your nerve cells are delicate and vulnerable to these environmental poisons, and our defense systems are not adapted to this particular fight. Designed to fend off the occasional poisonous mushroom or spoiled bit of food, the constant barrage of chemical neurotoxins overwhelms our detoxification systems, and nerve cells die.

High Cortisol

Just as stress-induced cortisol causes negative effects on your body, high cortisol also has a significant impact on your brain. High cortisol levels destroy the cells in your hippocampus, the part of your brain responsible for memory and learning. High cortisol along with high adrenaline levels also puts your brain in a heightened state of alertness, ready to fight or run. If this goes on for extended periods of time, we burn ourselves out and descend into a cortisol-mediated depression. In a similar vein, chronic pain leads to brain changes as well. The remarkable Stanford-based neuroscientist Robert Sapolsky has written extensively about this in his book *Why Zebras Don't Get Ulcers*, which I highly recommend reading.

Early-Childhood Trauma

Neuroscientists now use a new technology called functional MRI (FMRI) to get pictures of the brain centers and map out brain structure. Scientists have recently found that childhood trauma, such as sexual, physical, and mental/emotional abuse, changes the structure of the brain. This effect continues into adulthood in what amounts to an emotionally generated type of brain cell trauma that can lead to depression in childhood or later in life.

Addiction

Every time I give a lecture I ask the audience to raise a hand if they or someone in their immediate family suffers from an addiction problem. You'd be amazed how often everyone's hand goes up. I have deep compassion for people that suffer from addiction and am dedicated to helping them by providing the extra level of attention addiction requires. Of course we all want a healthy level of serotonin and dopamine in our synapses, bouncing around and hitting those light switches on our post-synaptic neurons. When your brain lights up, you feel good, alive, ready for anything. Unfortunately, drugs, such as alcohol, and even some foods can trigger addiction responses in the brain, causing changes in brain chemicals. This gives us a "boost," but when chemical levels drop back down we feel bad and want another drink, or another Oreo cookie.

Some people crave alcohol or foods because consuming them elevates what were previously low brain chemicals, while other people develop low brain chemicals by burning them out from overconsumption of alcohol or certain foods. The end result is the same: a complete dependence on a substance to keep the brain cells firing and a seeking/addictive behavior to assure that the brain gets the chemicals it needs.

3. GENETIC TYPE

In May of 2011 I attended a three-day conference called One Mind For Research, a gathering of 200 of the world's top neuroscientists brought together by Patrick Kennedy and Garen Staglin. Kennedy wanted the integrative neurology field to be represented, so I was invited. One of the highlights of the conference (which ended with a keynote speech from Vice President Biden) was the constant presence of Francis Collins, the researcher who led the Human Genome Project. Collins and his team solved one of the biggest scientific puzzles in human history, mapping out every gene in the human body. This knowledge has catapulted science forward to a place most neuroscientists could not even have fantasized about a generation ago. Genes regulate everything from the color of your eyes to the numbers of dopamine receptors in your brain. It's possible you are a Genetic Type, born with a broken brain rather than experiencing neurotransmitter depletion or nerve cell damage. Usually we can figure this out simply by examining your family tree and creating what's called a genogram, a map of every relative and what their physical and mental health problems were. If you see depression, schizophrenia, drug addiction, alcoholism, suicide, and so on sprinkled throughout the genogram, you can suspect genetics may be a factor. Ashley, age 12, her mom Karen, and her grandmother Judy provide a most striking example of this. Each of them has the exact same brain chemistry imbalance measured on the lab tests I use. Seeing the effects of low dopamine echo throughout each generation shows a trail of tragedy and human suffering that to me seems almost unbearable.

Why is Depression on the Rise?

The lines on charts depicting depression rates, from the Centers for Disease Control to the World Health Organization, point straight up. There is no doubt depression is increasing, and not just in the United States but also worldwide. It's already the number one cause of lost days of work and lost productivity, and if the trend continues, depression will outpace all other health problems in terms of both its economic and social costs. Why is depression on the rise? If you look at the underlying causes in the previous section of this chapter you can see clearly that besides bad genetics, the other issues that trigger depression are looming larger for us. From head wounds in our current wars where Kevlar armor keeps our soldiers' bodies protected but can't protect their brains, to an increase in environmental toxins, to the cumulative impact of poor nutrition and increased stress, all explain why we are hitting a crisis level of depression. Conventional psychiatrists scramble around looking for solutions, but orthodox medicine has very limited tools to bring to bear on this problem, given its scale and level of severity.

WHAT ARE THE CONVENTIONAL MEDICAL SOLUTIONS?

Psychotropic Medications

The pharmaceutical dart game is dangerous, because your brain functions as the dartboard which physicians toss darts at in the form of powerful, side effect prone drugs. These medications have become the primary treatment for depression. The original antidepressants were called tricyclics, and while still in use today, they have been mostly replaced by another class of drugs, SSRIs (selective serotonin reuptake inhibitors). No one really knows the exact mechanism of action of these drugs. We know they can work from watching how they impact people, but the exact science behind the mechanism remains a mystery. Later we'll discuss two competing theories about this.

Cognitive Behavioral Therapy

There's no question: Talking about your problems helps you feel better. Psychotherapy that is based on a system called Cognitive Behavioral Therapy has wonderful outcomes and helps relieve depression. It is grossly under-used now because of the focus on medications and pill-taking versus human interaction. Other forms of psychotherapy can also help, including group therapy, body-oriented therapy, emotional release work, and dozens of other techniques.

Electroconvulsive Therapy

Just seeing a picture of Jack Nicholson makes me want to crack up laughing. I love his movies. If you are old enough to remember his early film One Flew Over the Cuckoo's Nest, it put the practice of electroshock therapy on the map. Although you might think about ECT as a part of psychiatric history, it is still in use today and can be very helpful for major depression. Down and blue after a bitter breakup, would you seek out electroshock therapy? I hope not. ECT, like antidepressant medications, should be reserved for special cases of moderate or major depression.

Addressing Multiple Causes of Depression

If you've sought treatment for depression from an orthodox doctor, you know that it's surprisingly hard to get a complete assessment. While an individual physician may address one or two of the known causes, treatments end up fragmented most of the time. If you add up what would be needed for a complete evaluation, it would look something like this: psychiatrist for medications, psychologist for therapy, endocrinologist to check hormones, nutritionist for vitamin D, and so on. This discombobulated system with individual practitioners working without any integration rarely works as it should.

OTHER MOOD DISORDERS: ADD/ADHD, ANXIETY, AND BIPOLAR

ADD

Conventional ADD treatments revolve almost exclusively around Adderall and another prescription amphetamine you've probably heard of, Ritalin. These two names have become part of every school principal's vocabulary, as they're often given to students in an attempt to help them "focus" on their classwork.

Anxiety

Tapping on your wine glass, about to give a speech at your best friend's wedding, being anxious makes sense. Nervousness about activities outside your usual routine causes your brain to fire off strong signals. If you experience anxiety unrelated to what's happening around you, or if a small trigger causes an overblown reaction, conventional doctors will prescribe a series of drugs called benzodiazapines, or benzos for short. Some of their names you might be familiar with include Xanax, Ativan, and Valium. These drugs work on the calming neurotransmitter GABA and stifle anxiety, making you mellow regardless of what's happening around you.

Bipolar

Conventional treatments for bipolar disorder revolve around a complex array of medications. Since bipolar disorder causes manic "up" periods, followed by dark depressions on a down cycle, often the drug cocktails shoot for a wide variety of effects. Mood stabilizers (like lithium or the anti-convulsant Lamictal) prevent the extreme highs and lows, while anti-psychotics (like Abilify or Zyprexa) may be used as mood stabilizers. Also, standard antidepressants and the anti-anxiety benzos often enter into the mix. Psychiatrists face a big challenge to get the combination just right and keep the person from being too up or too down.

How Well Do Conventional Treatments Work?

You'll be shocked to learn how poorly these treatments work and how often they make people worse. In my top ten list of "must read" books, Julian Whitacre's *Anatomy of an Epidemic* describes the horrors in detail and points out the toll we pay for continuing to rely on harmful and ineffective treatments. Why is this happening? Mostly it's because conventional medicine has no other way of treating depression.

Short-Term Effects

Over the short-term, antidepressant medications provide some measurable level of relief to between 8-12% of the people that take them. That means 88-92% of people miss out on any benefits. The placebo effect, or what happens when patients are unknowingly given only a sugar pill, runs between 30-40% for depression. In other words, taking a fake pill helps 3 to 4 times more people than the real medications do. In people over age 65 the odds of getting a medication-based benefit drops from an average of 10% down to 0%. It gets worse. This small percentage of potential benefit has to be weighed against what we've talked about before, that antidepressants can, in the long-term, make people worse.

Long-Term Effects

While the short-term effects look unspectacular at best, the long-term effects are downright scary. Whitacre reviews many long-term outcome studies in his book, and there is no good news to be found. Long-term use of antidepressants leads to a higher risk of being depressed. Long-term use of ADD medications puts you at risk for developing bipolar disorder. Long-term use of bipolar treatments increases the odds you will experience more severe episodes. Long-term use of benzos creates addiction, and all of these classes of drugs cause long-standing changes to the structure and function of the brain. I am not completely against these types of medications, but you should be aware of the good and bad aspects of their use and make your treatment decisions based on a full understanding of their cost/ benefit analysis. Remember that the intended use of these drugs is for special cases of moderate to major depression. If you or a family member is seriously considering a psychiatric hospital or electroshock therapy, then these medications can make sense.

Outmoded Model of Depression: Monoamine Theory

If I said "heart disease," you'd say "high cholesterol." If I said "diabetes," you'd say "insulin." In a similar manner, if you say "depression" to conventional doctors, they'll say "serotonin." Modern medicine depicts depression as a serotonin-deficiency problem. The theory of serotonin causing depression came about through chance observation. In the 1950s while experimenting on tuberculosis patients, researchers stumbled on a drug that seemed to elevate the moods of some of the TB patients. This "happy" drug, called a tricyclic, was found to boost serotonin levels in the brain, so the common-sense theory was born that low levels of serotonin must be what make people unhappy or depressed. This theory is called the Monoamine Theory because serotonin is part of a class of chemicals called Monoamines. No one, however, has been able to prove this theory. In the next chapter I will cover the latest theory that explains depression's cause, called the Neuron Bundle Damage theory.

The Kalish Method and Conventional Treatments

Conventional science acknowledges that stress causes depression. As we discussed in detail earlier, the Kalish Method focuses on treating stress hormones as a foundation to healing the brain. Conventional medicine knows that neurotransmitters are involved in depression. In the Kalish Method this is acknowledged as well, and my work also addresses serotonin and dopamine problems, just using different techniques. We all agree low vitamin D can contribute to depression, but the Kalish Method incorporates the idea of getting outside and increasing exposure to sunlight, along with taking vitamin D supplements. For exercise, diet, and even hormone balancing, the Kalish Method treats the exact same problems substituting natural therapies for prescription drugs whenever possible and making medications the last resort rather than relying on them exclusively.

The incorporation of lifestyle changes; natural therapies; lab testing for stress hormones, female hormones, and brain chemicals; it all adds up and takes time and energy on your part. It's easier and more convenient to take a single pill of an antidepressant medication once a day. So just how much work does it take to get your brain healthy without relying on medications? I'll start to explain the details in Chapter Five.

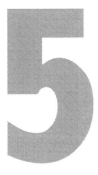

5

. . . .

HEALING THE MIND: A TEST-BASED MODEL FOR CORRECTING NT IMBALANCES

Introducing Dr. Marty Hinz

Imagine how excited orthopedic physicians were by the invention of the X-ray, as for the first time they could see the broken bones they were treating. Now what if I told you there's a way to map your mind, a way to peek inside your head and get an X-ray equivalent of your brain in action? No more guessing about what's happening, no more haphazard tossing of antidepressant darts called Zoloft, Prozac, Wellbutrin, or Celexa. When I first heard about this new technology I was suspicious. If valid, why wasn't this discovery front page news? The answer is because in the United States it's against the law to claim that any non-drug treatment can treat or "cure" a disease, so mind mapping remains under the radar.

The man who pioneered this revolutionary method is Marty Hinz, MD, a dedicated physician and researcher who spent the last 14 years focused on unraveling the mysteries of the mind. He has developed a method showing how serotonin and dopamine levels can be measured and then balanced to create a properly functioning brain. Producing this breakthrough in relative obscurity, and publishing research papers on his findings that mainstream medicine has ignored, Dr. Hinz's work needs to be made public. That's part of my mission in writing this book.

His amazing discovery began with a chance occurrence. Running his practice in Duluth, Minnesota for decades, Hinz created a medical weight-loss program to help his obese and diabetic patients lose weight. When the drug treatment he was using was taken off the market, these patients quickly gained the weight back, and their health problems returned: high blood pressure, diabetes, high cholesterol. Dr. Hinz became desperate to find another drug treatment for weight loss. He tried using a protocol with antidepressants, but achieved mixed results. He then made a crucial decision that would change the direction of his career and open an entirely new area of brain research.

Dr. Hinz tried something never attempted before in orthodox medicine. He gathered his biochemistry textbooks and pieced together the specific biochemical pathways for the production of serotonin and dopamine. Using his brilliant analytical mind, he unravelled the biochemistry of the brain. Just like creating a recipe, he laid out every ingredient the body uses to make the chemicals the brain requires to function properly.

Having been a conventional physician for decades, he now found himself in foreign territory, straying away from traditional medical rules and standards of care. He willingly exposed himself to potential criticism and ostracization from the medical boards. There were no drugs on the market that met his needs, so he trotted off to a local health food store in Duluth and put together his "brain cocktail" using nutritional supplements. The mix he created contained every single nutrient required to fuel the brain.

Never having recommended any type of supplementation before, Dr. Hinz began careful implementation of his new protocol. Weeks passed, and as his weight-loss patients followed the program, something incredible happened. Not only did his patients begin to lose weight again, but their blood pressures also improved, and his diabetic patients stabilized and regained control of their blood sugar levels. Impressed by the results, Hinz put more and more patients on his nutritional regimen.

Do you remember the "mood lifting" side effect of the experimental drugs given to tuberculosis patients, the drugs we now call antidepressants? The same dynamic now played out in Hinz's clinic in Duluth. Many patients reported an alleviation of their depressions, and migraine headaches they'd suffered from for years disappeared. People with fibromyalgia and body aches and pains began to feel better. These reports were so consistent among his patients taking the supplements that he began to realize he was on to something much bigger than a simple weight-loss program.

Introduction of Lab Testing

Hinz then took a second crucial step in this story. He set out to measure what the nutritional supplements were doing. Never having used supplements before, he needed data to verify what he was observing every day in his practice. Acquiring this data necessitated the development of lab tests. Neuroscientists had given up on measuring people's serotonin and dopamine levels because the early testing techniques showed no correlation between urine levels and brain levels of these chemicals. Blood tests were also abandoned because of what's called the blood brain barrier, which prevents serotonin and dopamine in the blood from entering the brain.

Undeterred by the previous failures of others, Hinz began measuring serotonin and dopamine levels in the urine of his patients. Past scientific literature showed high urinary serotonin levels in some people with depression, and low levels in others, with no discernible pattern. In other words, a person could be depressed regardless of their serotonin levels. Adding even more confusion, when previous researchers had looked at the impact of amino acids (the main nutrients Hinz was using with his patients) on serotonin levels, there was also no correlation found. People taking amino acids would sometimes have their urinary serotonin levels go up, and sometimes go down. There was no correlation established between the amino acids and the test results.

Hinz decided to continue his investigation in the same way Darwin began his study of evolution – with data collection. And not just by gathering data on 100 people for twelve weeks and immediately drawing conclusions like many drug trials do. Hinz wanted to collect massive amounts of data over many years. To accomplish this, he set up a system that linked medical clinics and gathered their lab-testing data on every patient into a single database, building up to a network of over 1,000 clinics.

A typical doctor in practice might see 50 weight-loss patients in a year, order 50 lab tests, and track 50 people's progress. Hinz created a system where he could look at 20,000 lab tests a year, eventually amassing a database with over 2.5 million patient days of data. No one had done this before, and that's why the potential benefits of testing urinary levels of these chemicals had been ignored for so long. Now with his massive database he began seeing trends and patterns that allowed him to solve the many riddles of neurotransmitter testing.

Studying the Kidneys, Studying the Brain

During this time Hinz also applied himself to the study of several seemingly unrelated areas. For two years he focused on nephrology, the study of the kidneys, and how the kidneys process the particular amino acids he was using with his program. During this time he discovered a series of obscure Italian research papers detailing every facet of the kidneys' use of amino acids. He then turned to the study of neurology, and the physiological mechanisms that control the brain. He saw that each piece in a never-before-assembled puzzle had been clearly laid out by scientists before him. The kidney specialists who looked at amino acids in the kidneys never thought about a possible link their work might have to the brain. Similarly, scientists studying the brain never thought to glance at the nephrology research literature, especially a topic as obscure as the kidneys' processing of amino acids supplied from supplements.

Dr. Marty Hinz looked at all the information and synthesized it. Finally he could explain what was in front of him the entire time.

Three Phase Model

How did every powerhouse research university in the neuroscience community miss what a humble family practitioner from Duluth discovered? Persistence, focus, and mounds and mounds of data made the difference. As I mentioned earlier, when Hinz first began testing people he found what had been seen previously: On a baseline test there is no relationship between urinary serotonin and dopamine levels and any condition worth investigating. Baseline testing was a complete dead end.

Stubborn, and you'd have to be to get through -40 degree winters, Hinz looked at what the testing showed with people in a treatment program. When people are tested while taking antidepressant medications, the same problem occurs as with baseline testing: There is no correlation with urine levels and anything else. At this point every previous researcher had given up. Hinz took it one step further. Based on the Italian medical research on the kidneys' processing of amino acids, he reasoned he could test people accurately if they were in a treatment program, but not one using conventional drugs. It would only work if he tested people while they took a fixed dose of amino acids. After that crucial adjustment, he began to see a very clear pattern emerging that no one had found before. When people take amino acids in certain fixed dosages, their urinary levels of serotonin and dopamine fall into what he called the "Three Phase Response." He published these findings much later in the journal *Neuropsychiatric Disease*

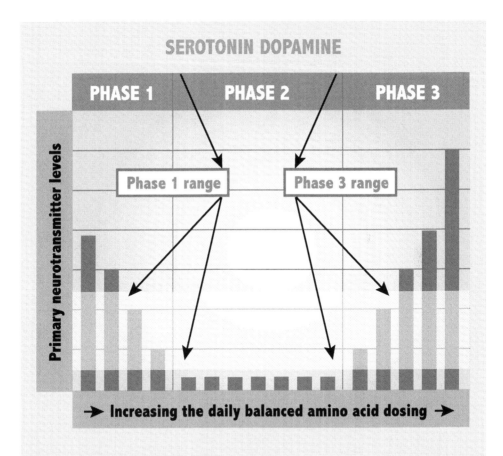

The discovery of three phases of urinary neurotransmitter levels was a breakthrough in understanding many decades of confusing scientific findings.

and Treatment in 2009, and again in more detail in 2010 in the journal *Reports and Research in Urology.*

With his Three Phase Response theory in hand, the past decades of previous findings now made sense. The data Hinz plotted mapped out a U-shaped curve. On the upper left-hand side of the U-curve was Phase

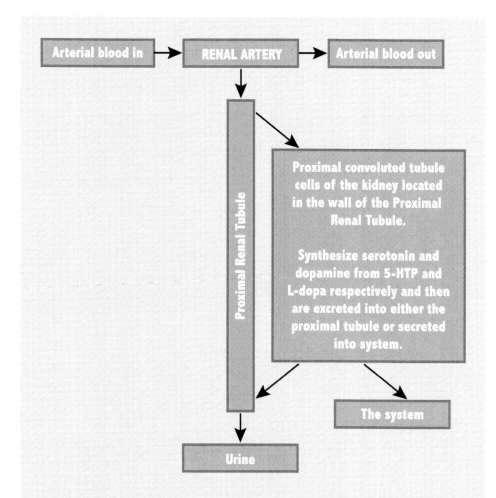

Your kidneys are busy making serotonin and dopamine all the time. So, the question is, are they going to dump them out in the urine or put them back into your body for you to use?

One, which shows high urinary levels of serotonin and dopamine occurring when these chemicals are dumped out of the kidneys into the urine. The bottom of the U-curve he called Phase 2, which shows low urine levels as the kidneys dump out less of these chemicals into the urine and the body holds on to more of them. Finally, Phase 3 describes the right side of the U-curve where levels are going up again in response to taking amino acids, as the body builds its levels and then dumps out the excess it doesn't need.

He now had a clear understanding of the urinary tests and how to get accurate results. The next major hurdle Hinz had to overcome was understanding how the urinary levels of serotonin and dopamine produced in the kidneys related to what was happening in the brain. Hinz knew that the kidneys contain organic cation transporters (OCT2s), little gates which serotonin and dopamine run through. Just like a gate going to a backyard, these OCT2 transporters can be closed (which blocks serotonin from entering the body), partially open, or fully open (allowing serotonin to flood into the body). It turns out that the Italian kidney physiology researchers had learned how this system works, leaving it up to Hinz to apply these concepts to his growing database of patients tested while taking amino acids.

The Three Phase Model works like this: When the OCT2 gates close, serotonin is dumped out in the urine and less comes into the body, causing urine test levels to be high. When partially open, serotonin rushes into the body and urine levels drop, since less is being dumped out. This makes the test levels low. When the gates are wide open, serotonin floods into the body and any excess spills out into the urine. This makes levels high again, just like when the gates are closed. The goal of treatment is to open the gates fully for both serotonin and dopamine so they can flood into your body and, ultimately, your brain.

Then came the final breakthrough, which pulled all the pieces together into one neat model. Hinz focused on the brain and how the OCT2 gates operate inside the head. It turns out that all mammals, from mice to humans, have identical gates in the kidneys and in the brain. These gates allow the movement of serotonin and dopamine in these two areas to occur in the exact same ways in the exact same moments. This syncing up of the kidney gates with the brain gates means we can measure the gate position in the kidneys with a non-invasive urine test and use this result to unlock precisely what is happening in the brain at that precise moment.

Now Hinz had a complete picture. When you are taking fixed dosages of amino acids, what is happening in the kidneys mimics exactly what is happening in the brain. The mind mapping process was complete. He could now measure and correct any serotonin or dopamine problems with precision.

The crucial roles of serotonin and dopamine

Serotonin and dopamine generate our moods and feelings, and even our sense of appetite. They are key components in creating our minds and thoughts and ultimately who we think we are. As Dr. Hinz learned early on, when levels of these brain chemicals are balanced, the appetite shrinks, a buzz of energy and a sense of well-being is created, and even body aches and pains dissipate.

Classified as an excitatory neurotransmitter, low dopamine levels lead to physical exhaustion and profound fatigue. If you are low in dopamine, just reading a book can be a struggle. Motivation and energy systems plummet. Low dopamine also causes concentration problems and various body symptoms, from body aches and pains to restless leg syndrome and tremors. The most severe manifestation of dopamine-related problems is Parkinson's disease, which I'll cover in detail later.

Serotonin, called an inhibitory neurotransmitter, calms us down. If serotonin levels are low, we get anxious, have trouble sleeping, have panic attacks, and experience neck and shoulder tension that won't go away. Low serotonin can also trigger digestive problems since the gut contains 95% of the serotonin in the body. Of course both low serotonin and low dopamine lead to depression.

Ultimately it's the balance of the two chemicals that keeps you healthy. People who have used this protocol routinely experience a wide variety of problems clearing up, including ADD, OCD, memory problems, migraines, fibromyalgia, and female hormone issues like hot flashes and night sweats.

Mind Mapping

With CT scans, PET scans, MRIs, and FMRIs, we can take a picture of the brain. Mind mapping allowed Dr. Hinz to get a virtual X-ray image of the mind. Can you think of anything more amazing? His process allows us to "see" into the brain and tell exactly which chemicals are low and what needs to be done to bring them back up using amino acid supplementation. Now anyone, regardless of how depleted they may be, can test their brain chemicals and use amino acids to balance them. Now that they can be measured, they can be fixed without guesswork.

Hinz has given us a powerful science-based method for treating the brain. Regardless of the source of the brain problem, this technique can be used to help restore normal function. If you have a deficiency issue, we will rebuild your levels and you'll feel better. If you have damage from trauma (like TBI) or chemical toxins (like Parkinson's), we will increase your levels high enough to restore normal firing. Even if you have a lifelong genetic issue with low brain chemicals, this same program can get your brain in gear again and get you feeling better than you ever have before.

Before insulin, diabetes meant certain death, and people only lived a couple of years. Scientists struggled for over fifty years to figure out how to treat diabetes, and now thanks to their efforts you can stroll into any drug store and get a glucose monitor and fill a prescription for insulin. A well-managed diabetic can test and correct their blood sugar daily and live a long, productive life. We have now reached the same point with the brain. Struggling for solutions since the 1950s, we now have the "insulin" we need. We have the test technology and the treatments, and certainly we have plenty of people who need help. My hope is that this book starts the ball rolling until amino acid brain treatments are as easy to get as treatment for diabetes.

I don't want to give anyone false hope, as these programs don't work for everyone. But if you have lots of negative thoughts, loss of motivation, lack of concentration, constantly feel tired, or find yourself overeating too often, when you begin one of Dr. Hinz's programs the odds are greatly in your favor that your life will change. Your thoughts will change. Most of the negativity will ease and you'll feel happy. The darkness disappears. The clouds go away. I watch this happen to people in my practice every day.

REVISITING PHASE ONE
OF THE KALISH PROTOCOL

I wish one day I could somehow capture and share all that I've been privileged to experience in the treatment room, especially the people I've worked with and their amazing stories of healing. I spend my work day fluctuating between admiring the tenacity and strength of the people I see, and being awestruck from watching the healing powers of the human body. If we can step out of the way and remove the blocks that restrict us, healing comes through like a river bursting through a dam. As I move forward in my career, I'm heading more in the direction of treating the brain, but I have found that it's still critical to treat the body. A healthy person is in a much better position to have a happy brain. We want people to be both healthy AND happy, first making sure the body is right, and then the mind.

This chapter is devoted to healing the body, and then in Chapter Seven we address healing the mind.

Healing the Body: What Causes the Big Five

Think back to a period in your life when you were under great emotional stress. A loved one died, or was diagnosed with cancer. You ended a long-term relationship, or your marriage ended. You went through a financial crisis, or were going full-time to school and working odd jobs. For most of you reading this book, your most serious health problems likely started within a year or two of a high-stress stretch of life.

Kristin had all of the Big Five symptoms. She was tired, slightly overweight, depressed, had heartburn periodically, and suffered from dramatic hormone-related mood swings. Her problems started when she was going to school full-time at a graduate program in creative writing while working full-time at a magazine. She was nearly finished with two years of 60-80 hour work weeks when she went to the Bahamas for her best friend's wedding. She picked up a stomach bug on the trip and never felt the same after that.

Kristin lived out a pattern you may have experienced also. Lots of pressures in your life cause your stress hormone levels to shoot up, and with the constant stress your immune system gets weaker. Off you go on a trip, whether it's to the Bahamas or to the local salad bar, and you pick up a digestive tract infection. Time goes by and eventually this low-grade digestive problem weakens your liver detox pathways, and you become prone to picking up the Big Five. This is the three key body systems collapsing one after the other.

What health issues bother you? When did they very first start? If you trace them back all the way, often to many years ago, how stressed out were you at that time? Were you like Kristin, overloaded with stress from having too much on your plate? I find that 95% of the people that walk into our clinic, just like Kristin, have stress as the key contributor or initiator of their current health problems.

Three Sources of Stress: Emotional, Dietary, Inflammatory

Stress hormone problems come from three main sources: emotional stress, dietary stress, or inflammatory stress. These three accumulate, all dumping into the same shared bucket, and when enough stress builds up, the bucket tips over and the symptoms spill out. Throughout our lives the biggest stresses usually come from emotions; if you have experienced the death of someone you love, or gone through a divorce, I'm sure you know exactly what I mean.

Little stresses can add up too. Dietary stress plays out in subtle ways every day with blood sugar control. If you skip breakfast, eat refined sugar, or eat carbs without any protein, you will throw off your blood sugar level, and two hormones, insulin and cortisol, will fight to balance things out. Each moment your blood sugar remains unstable your body suffers, although you probably won't feel it happening at the time. This dietary stress accumulates and builds up over the years. After one such dietary faux pas mentioned above, insulin takes sugar from the blood and puts it into fat cells. Cortisol then cranks up to bring blood sugar levels back to normal. Have a muffin and coffee for breakfast, and you'll be on a blood sugar hormone roller coaster the rest of the day and into the evening, storing body fat and craving sugar. The detailed diet advice to help you solve this issue is on page 148 of this book. The abbreviated version is: Eat within an hour of waking up, always include protein with each meal, don't ever skip meals, and keep portion sizes small (no supersizing). If you need extra support, include two small snacks, one midmorning and one midafternoon.

The third category of stress on your body is inflammation. You may already be aware of your inflammation, or it can be hidden. If you have arthritis, tendonitis, bursitis, gastritis, colitis, or any condition with an *itis* at the end, then you have known *inflammation*. The suffix *itis* means inflamed, so arthritis means "inflamed joints," colitis means "inflamed colon," and so on. You could also have hidden inflammation in your body that you don't notice on a day-to-day basis. If your knees are swollen and painful, then it's no mystery that you have arthritis in your knees. But if your small intestine becomes inflamed every time you eat gluten, you may have absolutely no idea something bad is happening. Most of us have some type of hidden inflammation, and that's what functional medicine lab assessments excel at: finding the source of hidden inflammation that must be removed for your body to heal.

Body Breakdown

Once exposed to enough stress from these three different areas – emotional, dietary, and inflammatory stressors – your body starts to break down. Ken worked extremely hard as an executive in New York City. Every weekday for 22 years he was in the gym at 5 a.m., then straight to his office, and back home in bed by midnight. By age 40, fifteen years into his personal experiment on human tolerance for enduring stress, his body started to break down and he became physically exhausted. He found himself just going through the motions at work and catching colds and flus constantly. He continued working, got used to be being sick most of the time, and took antibiotics constantly until he turned 47 and realized he didn't have much of a life left anymore as he sniffled and hacked his way through the days.

I tested and corrected Ken's stress hormones, and after about a year of working together with both nutritional supplement programs and lifestyle changes, his immune system came back on line, his energy returned to what it was like in college, and his excitement about work rekindled, albeit now at a more sustainable pace. Ken's story is emblematic of what I see in many people I work with. Many of you will likely suffer through 10-15 years of low-level symptoms, gradually getting worse and worse until finally your body breaks down enough that you're finally forced to get help.

Jenny is a 35-year-old who worked with the diplomatic corps and had many years under her belt in overseas assignments. Her depression and fatigue and PMS-related mood swings started after a trip to Guatamala and were getting worse each year. It reached the point where she was missing work at least a week every month just before her period, forced to stay home incapacitated.

With Jenny we ran the exact same lab tests as with Ken. The beauty of functional medicine comes through in that it's not symptom based. In other words, with the Kalish Method we order the same tests regardless of where you stand symptom-wise, because the model says one or more of the three key body systems most likely has broken down and that the symptoms result from this breakdown. We don't treat symptoms, we treat the three key body systems. This greatly simplifies the diagnostic portion of my job. I run a lab test for each body system and fix what I find using natural therapies. It's that straightforward.

To give you a sense of how this works, to test the adrenal glands we measure cortisol and DHEA, to test digestive health we check for food reactions and low-grade infections in the digestive tract, and we measure your liver detox pathways by checking for specific nutrients that help your body dump out toxins. Let's take a look at each of these body systems in turn.

Adrenal Function (Cortisol and Stress)

Stress hormones such as cortisol literally "fry" brain cells, and balancing cortisol is part of setting the foundation for a healthy body and a healthy brain. People know that stress impacts their health, but I think most of us feel powerless to do anything about it. As cortisol levels burn out and adrenal function diminishes, you get tired. You reach a level of exhaustion that seems constant, unrelieved by rest or sleep. If cortisol drops more, then you might start to feel depressed too. The things that used to be fun aren't anymore. You might come home after work and just feel like doing nothing instead of meeting up with friends or interacting with your kids. Going to the gym or seeing a movie seems like a chore or a burden now. Check out the Stress Questionnaire on page 173 and see how much of it applies to you.

FOUR LIFESTYLE CHANGES TO REDUCE ADRENAL STRESS

Lifestyle changes make up the core of adrenal repair programs and you can start with any one of the four: diet, exercise, sleep, or stress management.

1. Diet

The diet to follow is a gluten-free and blood sugar control diet. Keep it simple at first by eliminating gluten. If that seems like too much for you

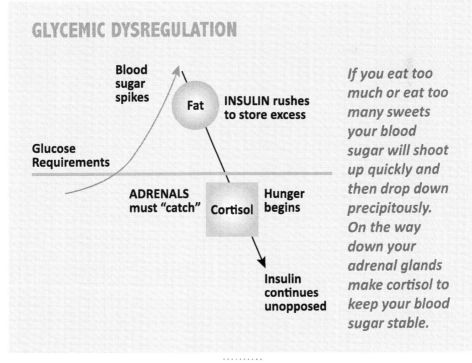

GLYCEMIC DYSREGULATION

Blood sugar spikes

Fat

INSULIN rushes to store excess

Glucose Requirements

ADRENALS must "catch"

Cortisol

Hunger begins

Insulin continues unopposed

If you eat too much or eat too many sweets your blood sugar will shoot up quickly and then drop down precipitously. On the way down your adrenal glands make cortisol to keep your blood sugar stable.

right now, then skip that step and begin by controlling your blood sugar. We can deal with the gluten issue later on.

2. Exercise

Most people in adrenal burnout want to exercise but don't have the energy for it. If you do have the energy, then start with 30 minutes a day, five days a week, and build up to 60 minutes a day over the course of several months. If you don't have a strong background in exercise and aren't sure what to do, then I highly recommend using a personal trainer. It's pretty much impossible to design your own exercise program unless you have some help. The CHEK Institute program's certified trainers (chekinstitute. com) are a good resource. If getting a trainer isn't financially realistic for you, then start with something easy that you can be sure won't hurt, like walking, yoga, swimming, or cycling. If you have an injury or problem that prevents you from these kinds of activities, then I would suggest going to a yoga class with a teacher that has a strong therapeutic background. Don't push yourself too hard, and if you can't figure out how to incorporate regular exercise right away, then work on the other three lifestyle changes and come back to this one later.

3. Sleep

What's the magic pill that helps heal everything, functional medicine's fountain of youth? What treatment can fix immune problems, fatigue, even weight gain? Every condition you can imagine can be improved with nature's original cure-all tonic, sleep. Sleep isn't something you get around to when you can fit it in. It is the essential component in healing. It's easy to cut back on sleep and feel like you are getting away with it, and as adults we don't recognize what happens from sleep deprivation, but it's quite clear if we look at what happens with little kids.

One summer when my son Asa was five years old we thought it would be fun to let him stay up to see the 4th of July fireworks. He didn't get to sleep until past 11 p.m. What happened? He turned into a monster for the next several days. A sleep-deprived five-year-old gets cranky and irritable, craves sugar, and becomes prone to emotional outbursts, behavioral problems at school, concentration problems in kindergarten class, and will likely get sick with some bug before you know it. What if we had kept him up until 11 p.m. for an entire month?

The important thing to know is that adults are no different. Without eight hours of uninterrupted deep sleep, you'll end up feeling and acting out just like an exhausted five-year-old. No difference whatsoever. You'll get cranky and have mood swings, crave sweets, have trouble focusing, and eventually get sick with some low-grade digestive tract infection. Remember from the previous section that adrenal exhaustion weakens the immune system and makes us prone to picking up bugs. It happens with little kids when they get tired, and it happens with adults too. No exceptions.

Any healing program you may attempt falters without adequate sleep. Remember, "Early to bed, early to rise, makes you healthy, wealthy, and wise." Your health, your ability to work effectively, and your brain all depend on sleep, and your biological clock, which is regulated by cortisol, dictates the timing of your sleep. Cortisol peaks at 6 a.m. in the morning, when you are designed to wake up, and cortisol drops lowest at 10 p.m., when you ideally should be falling asleep. The further from this natural clock you stray and the later after 10 p.m. you stay awake, the more compromised your system becomes.

4. Stress Management

Jerry, a gifted and dedicated surgeon, began working with me. He didn't think he had any current health problems; he just wanted to keep it that way. Given his line of work, every day Jerry saw in the operating room what happens when we ignore self-care over the years. As we sat down and went through his lifestyle factors, I discovered he worked 120 hours a week, which to be honest I didn't know was even possible. He put in over 80 hours a week in surgery, had at least 30 hours a week of administrative duties since he was the head of his department, and he spent an additional 10-12 hours a week in his role as president of a national surgical association.

After I got over my disbelief and absorbed what Jerry's week was like, we spent the rest of the session sorting through his work duties and carving out a more reasonable schedule. He had started off as a surgeon expected to temporarily perform 80 hour work weeks, but as he progressed professionally new duties kept piling up. He didn't want to let his surgical team members down and slack off on what he saw as his fair share of the patient load, so he tried to do it all. By the time we met he was basically working the equivalent of three full-time jobs. Jerry's healing program included supplements based on his adrenal lab tests, but the primary "treatment" was creating time for him to exercise and sleep more which he accomplished by turning over some of his surgical duties to the younger physicians working under him. Lifestyle coaching in the area of stress management for people like Jerry becomes the critical factor for determining the success of their health plan.

Adrenal Lab Tests

The moment I got a look at my new patient Keri's adrenal test results, I picked up the phone and got her scheduled to come in. Keri's cortisol was sky-high, and we needed to work together to improve this right away. Using an individualized lab-based supplement program, Keri's high cortisol was under control in a little over two months. Her panic attacks and anxiety faded, and her libido returned. Another patient, Stu, was just the opposite. He had incredibly low cortisol levels. He was so exhausted he could barely get out of bed in the morning, and he crashed again as soon as he got home from work. He had stopped seeing friends during the week, was achy all over, and just didn't feel well. His program took much longer to kick in, but after about six months he woke up one day and realized he really was better. It had been such a gradual process that he hadn't perceived any sudden changes, but month by month his energy came back, his joint pain receded, and at the end of the process he realized how far he had come.

Keri and Stu required nearly opposite treatment programs to shift their adrenals. To lower her cortisol, Keri desperately needed specific nutrients, like phosphorylated serine, magnesium, and calcium, along with adrenal hormone supports like DHEA and pregnenolone. Stu needed the exact opposite: a building up of low cortisol which we achieved with licorice root extract, blood sugar support nutrients, and adaptagenic herbs like ginseng, rhodiola, and ashwagandha. The programs I design use certain supplements to replace what you may be deficient in and use others to get your internal production of cortisol back to normal as quickly as possible. Once you are back on track the supplements stop and your body will take over, again self-manufacturing proper levels of cortisol as it should.

If you have significant adrenal hormone issues, then the odds favor your also having developed problems with Body System Two, the digestive system.

DIGESTIVE HEALTH: DIET AND PATHOGENS

Gluten-Free

I was at a restaurant in Dallas recently, and before I could order, the waitress started giving me a mini-lecture about their gluten-free menu and why gluten-free was so important. I wanted to say something along the lines of, "I was using gluten-free diets before you were even born," which was probably true, but I ended up just nodding and politely ordering fish tacos for dinner (with corn tortillas). Years ago when Dr. Timmins first taught me about gluten-free eating, gluten-free was little known. It seemed strange and off-putting, and came across as a bit contrary. To follow the Kalish Method's basic flow, when your adrenal stress hormones remain high and your digestive tract wears down, you become more prone to reacting to gluten. This same wear and tear process also sets the stage for picking up infections in your digestive tract.

This sequence I keep mentioning turns out to be the key to understanding many of your health problems and bears repeating because it's so common and so rarely recognized. These systems feed back and forth. The adrenals' degeneration triggers gut problems and food reactions, and digestive bugs need to be corrected to ensure proper nutrient absorption and to reduce inflammation, both essential elements for normal adrenal function. Do you have digestive symptoms like gas, bloating, heartburn, constipation, or diarrhea? About 95% of the time these common issues of the tummy resolve with a well-constructed functional medicine treatment program.

If you suspect gluten is an issue, page 39 has a gluten questionnaire you can fill out to see what your risk of this problem is. I also have a blood sugar questionnaire on page 170 to help you tease out that particular problem. Most of you will find that a gluten-free diet that also maintains your blood sugar will get your adrenals and digestion back on track in two to six weeks. If this isn't enough to fix the problem, you might need to take additional gut repair supplements. Gluten and blood sugar can also be screened for with a conventional blood test, which is well worth doing if you have access to a doctor who can order one for you.

Pathogens

Ron and Patricia were taking their dream vacation in Africa, and while traveling down the Nile in river rafts they were both dumped out in rough water. Unfortunately, and with extremely bad timing, that part of the river had a raw sewage spill, and they were both swimming in what amounted to an expansive, swirling toilet. They returned to the U.S. and immediately visited my clinic; both tested positive for parasites. It's hard to know what the real statistics may be, but for the people I test, about 75% have at least one parasite.

Intestinal parasites, along with bacteria and yeast overgrowth, block your absorption of nutrients in the digestive tract, lowering your overall nutritional status and making you prone to any one of the Big Five. This also deprives your adrenal glands, liver detox pathways, and brain of the key nutrients they require. To remedy this I test everyone I can for gastrointestinal infections. People aren't thrilled with this part as it involves collecting a stool sample, not exactly a crowd pleaser. But the results you experience in terms of improved health are well worth those challenging moments when you are scooping your poop.

Liver Detox Pathways

Once your adrenals implode, and your gut gets involved, these events add up and your liver detox pathways become strained. Ideally, liver detox pathways break down and remove harmful substances from the body. If this system gets backed up and toxins increase, you might start to notice skin problems, allergies, or a general malaise.

Page 175 has the questionnaire to figure out how toxic you may be. These toxins surround us, from car exhaust to nail polish remover, from your dental fillings to the pesticides sprayed on food. You should "go green" and make an effort to avoid toxins as much as possible. Buy non-toxic household cleaners, air purifiers, and shower filters to keep your home safe. Drink two or three quarts of filtered water every day, eat organic foods, and use chemical-free beauty care products to keep your body safe. Why does this matter so much? These toxins build up in your body and cause serious problems when they enter your brain tissue and start to damage nerve cells. This build up of toxins from your liver's failure to detoxify rapidly enough causes the neuron damage I spoke about in Chapter Five.

In the next chapter we'll look more specifically at brain-related conditions that can occur from nerve cell damage.

7

THE KALISH METHOD FOR DEPRESSION, ANXIETY, AND FATIGUE

Mind Mapping

I was very skeptical when I saw my first neurotransmitter test. I used a popular lab company and the results they returned made no sense. The supplement program recommendations seemed more like a multi-level marketing scheme than a science-based health program, and I was turned off. Fortunately, several years later a colleague told me about a different neurotransmitter lab company, Neuroresearch. He said they had a huge amount of data behind their protocols without the marketing hype. I ordered my first test from Neuroresearch, and later saw an ad for a Neuroresearch seminar in my hometown of San Francisco. I went out of curiosity, still somewhat cynical and not expecting much.

To my great surprise, at that weekend seminar I gained an appreciation of the brain and how to treat brain disorders. I have developed a genuine passion for perfecting this system of mapping the mind. I also found a mentor in Dr. Hinz, and a vast new area to study. Mind mapping opens up a whole new realm of lab-based treatments for brain disorders, and this chapter shows how these programs work.

Depression, Anxiety, and Fatigue

It's against the law in the United States to claim to "treat" depression with anything other than medications or surgery. As a natural health practitioner, I'd go to jail if I had a sign saying, "Get your depression treatments here." Not just a semantic argument to avoid liability, mind mapping doesn't "treat" depression or anxiety in the traditional sense of the word. In functional medicine we put our focus on lab tests and nutritional interventions that restore normal function and normal physiology, and restoring normal biochemistry isn't really a "treatment." It's a process of making things normal, not an intervention per se. If your depression goes away when you have normal serotonin and dopamine levels, then so be it.

"Treating" specific "conditions" doesn't fit in with the functional medicine model, and as you've already seen, in functional medicine we don't get overly wrapped up with specific symptoms and we try to avoid "this for that" type treatments. Examples of "this for that" type treatments are taking antidepressants for depression, or anti-anxiety medications for anxiety. Instead, functional medicine practitioners suggest that you lose weight, begin exercising, and get your cortisol and brain chemicals balanced to restore normal body functions. Your depression will then improve on its own, but the treatment comes from a combination of lifestyle changes and natural solutions.

Anxiety falls into the same category as depression. Low serotonin can trigger panic attacks and anxiety, so when your serotonin and dopamine levels are balanced using amino acids, the anxiety can be alleviated. This "treatment" is based on a complete analysis of the entire neurotransmitter system and a correction of that entire system. No "this for that" type treatment, it's not a case of, for example, 5-HTP supplementation preventing anxiety, as that would be treating a medical condition with a supplement. Once again, rather than "this supplement treats that condition," the goal of the brain work is to restore normal physiology and see the results. Thankfully it turns out that when your brain chemicals become balanced, many symptoms clear up quickly.

Fatigue comes in many forms. Some of you may be so exhausted you don't want to go to work, or even leave the house. Others may be tired

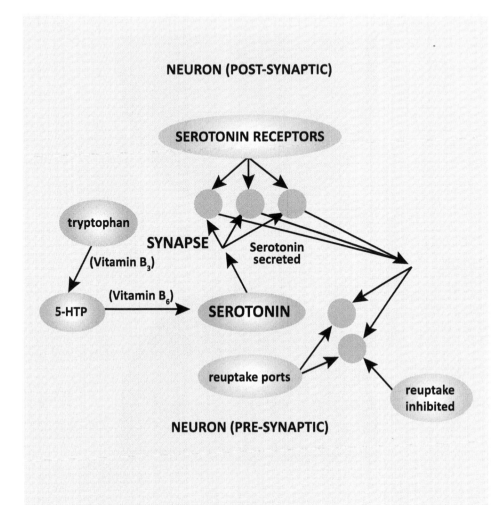

Your brain cells can only make serotonin from 5-HTP. All medications used to manipulate serotonin change its location, not the amount you make.

after exercising or eating too many carbs. Again, as with depression and anxiety, no specific "treatment" exists for fatigue in the mind mapping system. We test and correct. We strive for a balance of the entire system. Our mantra is, "Restore normal function, restore normal function," over and over, from condition to condition. This systems-based approach works well for many problems, including fatigue, which often clears up as dopamine levels improve.

How This Works

The brain-repair programs use the amino acids 5-HTP and tyrosine along with cofactors to increase brain activity, and then simple urine tests taken weekly to determine your ideal levels. Simple on the surface, the depth of the science behind the mind-mapping process stuns me. Billions of brain cells physically generate your thoughts and feelings, like a projector at a movie house generates a film you become immersed in. Let's take a

SYNTHESIS

If you give 5-HTP alone, serotonin levels increase, but this stimulates an increase in the enzyme that helps increase serotonin. This will also increase dopamine synthesis from tyrosine, which in the beginning may relieve symptoms. But if 5-HTP is administered over long periods of time, dopamine will be depleted unless tyrosine is also supplemented. The reverse is also true; using tyrosine alone will lower serotonin.

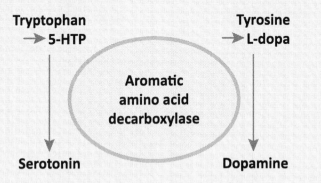

Using a single amino acid like 5-HTP will boost serotonin levels and may relieve many symptoms, but over time dopamine levels will rise also, and then dopamine will become depleted and an imbalance will occur.

moment and look behind the scenes and see how this movie we call your mind is made.

The Three Phase Model

In Chapter Five I discussed The Three Phase Model in detail. Now we can talk about how this applies to you. As a quick review, Phase One is when your urine levels of brain chemicals remain high as your body spills out or excretes these compounds rather than holding on to them. Phase Two is when your "gates" open and neurotransmitters rush into your body, reducing the amount measured in the urine on the test but increasing the amount available for your brain to use. Finally, in Phase Three your transporters (or "gates") become saturated, so full that the excess neurotransmitters get dumped in the urine. Just like in Phase One, your urinary levels look high, but now the opposite from Phase One occurs inside your brain, as your brain levels of these chemicals have elevated to where we want them to be.

Getting both serotonin and dopamine in a Phase Three response at the same time means we have achieved the best brain function possible. I hope each of you gets to experience what this feels like. Even though I have witnessed hundreds of people going through this process, it defies description. Life-long depression, anxiety, and long-term fatigue clear up in weeks. Almost like a magic trick, when the brain successfully resets, so many body functions improve that I am shocked each day in my clinic as I see these stories play out. It's challenging to get to this point because what is done to boost up one brain chemical impacts the other in a seesaw, back and forth pattern that can prove frustrating during the testing process. This chaos can be explained by the dual-gate lumen model.

Dual-Gate Lumen Model

The dual-gate lumen model sounds like double talk but explains much of what you will see on your tests as serotonin and dopamine levels bounce around like two 4-year-olds on a trampoline. If one kid stands on the trampoline and the other kid jumps up and down, the kid standing will get tossed around. Similarly, if serotonin goes up, dopamine can go up or down. If dopamine goes up, serotonin can also shift either up or down.

TRANSPORT (UPTAKE AND SECRETION)

The amino acid precursors tyrosine, L-dopa, tryptophan, and 5-HTP, along with the neurotransmitters serotonin, dopamine, norepinephrine, and epinephrine, are filtered at the glomerulous, then via the cation uptake ports are actively transported into the proximal convoluted renal tubule cells (PCRTC).

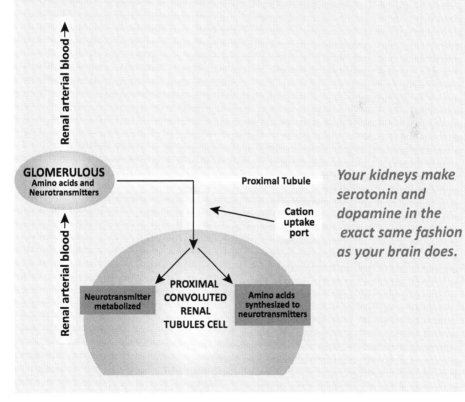

Renal arterial blood →

GLOMERULOUS
Amino acids and
Neurotransmitters

Renal arterial blood →

Proximal Tubule

Cation
uptake
port

Neurotransmitter
metabolized

**PROXIMAL
CONVOLUTED
RENAL
TUBULES CELL**

Amino acids
synthesized to
neurotransmitters

Your kidneys make serotonin and dopamine in the exact same fashion as your brain does.

Making sense of this seemingly random movement was one of Dr. Hinz's major breakthroughs.

In Hinz's 2010 article in the *Journal of Neuropsychiatric Disease and Treatment* he outlined for the first time this new picture of how the

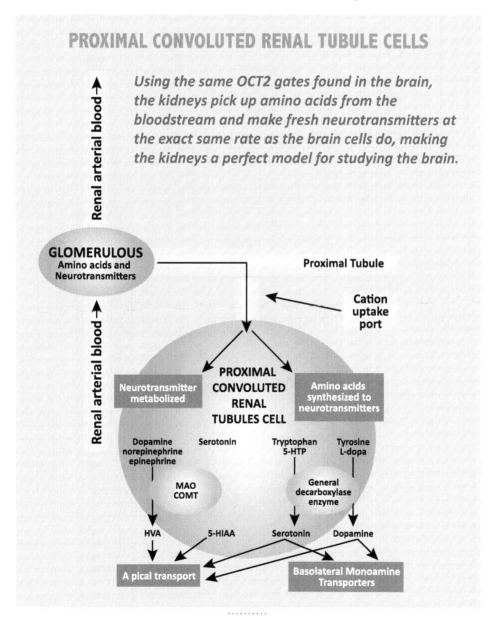

kidneys work, based on 75,000 lab results from over 7,500 different people (we'll get back to the brain in a minute). In the picture below you can see the dual-gate lumen model. Both serotonin and dopamine have their own gates. Imagine the subway system in New York, where turnstiles (gates) sit side by side and people line up to get through one of the gates. We have two "gates" in the kidneys, one that allows serotonin to go through, and one for dopamine. These gates can operate completely independently.

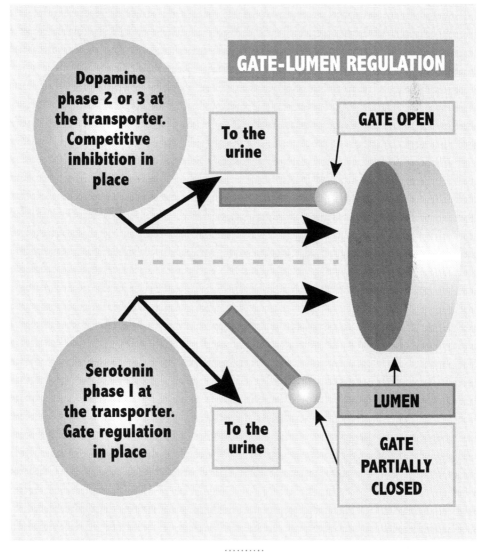

GATE-LUMEN REGULATION

Dopamine phase 2 or 3 at the transporter. Competitive inhibition in place

To the urine

GATE OPEN

Serotonin phase I at the transporter. Gate regulation in place

To the urine

LUMEN

GATE PARTIALLY CLOSED

This means you could have serotonin surging into your body through one gate while its neighboring dopamine gate remains stuck closed.

The goal of treatment is to get both gates open and "saturated," or full of neurochemicals, at the same time. One more important fact about the kidneys is that they filter serotonin and dopamine from the blood stream, pulling them out and breaking them down into individual amino acids. Therefore, the amounts of serotonin or dopamine in the blood bears no relationship to the amounts found in the urine. What is seen on lab results turns out to be the serotonin and dopamine newly made in the kidneys in response to how much of the amino acids tyrosine and 5-HTP have been taken in. The more tyrosine and 5-HTP obtained from supplements, the more serotonin and dopamine the kidneys make. You can see the importance of this because now we have an exact correlation: Amino acids go up (from the supplements taken), and serotonin and dopamine in the urine go up. It is that simple. And now for the brain part: The beauty of this system comes from scientific literature that shows that the gates in the kidneys mimic exactly what the gates in the brain are doing. This means that the urine testing shows, indirectly, precisely what is occurring in the brain. The map of kidney function can serve as an exact map of brain function.

Many obstacles made this connection unclear to generations of researchers, one being that the blood brain barrier keeps the serotonin and dopamine in the blood out of the brain. So blood levels do not correlate with urinary levels or with what is happening in the brain. This prevented scientists from developing an accurate picture of the urinary testing results for decades.

Neuron Bundle Damage Theory

Because antidepressant medications seem to act by boosting neurotransmitter levels in the synapse, it has been assumed that a low level of brain chemicals causes depression. What if this is wrong? What would it change? Certainly it would change our thinking about why depression rates keep rising. This part of the depression story is quite interesting because no one has ever proven that low serotonin causes depression; as mentioned before, that has been an assumption based on how various drugs work. Now that a massive database exists, with measurements of tens of thousands of people's levels of serotonin and other neurotransmitters mapped out, we actually know what is happening. There is no relationship between low serotonin and depression. Some depressed people have normal serotonin levels, and others don't. Some people have low serotonin and show no signs of depression whatsoever. The level of serotonin in the brain does not correlate with depression. So what does?

It turns out that neuron bundle damage does. A neuron bundle refers to a bunch of individual neurons bound together, like a rope made up of individual strands of fiber knitted together. Neurons get damaged from either physical trauma (head injury) or chemical trauma (neurotoxin exposure). A healthy neuron bundle can fire fully. A damaged neuron bundle, however, loses its firing capacity; if half the neurons have been destroyed, then the firing capacity is reduced by 50%. Let's say, for example, that in a healthy brain it takes 100 units of serotonin to allow 100 nerve cells in a nerve bundle to all fire and conduct signals properly. Well, if half those nerve cells were inoperable, you would need 200 units of serotonin to get the viable cells to create the effect of a normally functioning neuron bundle. By getting these healthy cells to do double duty (by firing twice as fast), you can help the damaged nerve bundle behave more like a healthy brain.

Neuron bundle damage theory may someday replace the current thinking of depression being a low-serotonin state. Boosting serotonin can help, but perhaps it is due to the neurons themselves being damaged, rather than the person having low serotonin. This does explain why depression would be on the rise worldwide: Rather than a sudden drop in worldwide serotonin levels, we just have more and more neurons being damaged from the increase in environmental toxins. Just like we have changed the physical environment by burning fossil fuels, leading to global warming, we have changed the internal environment inside the brain, loading it up with neurotoxins that kill brain cells.

Organic Cation Transporters and Competitive Inhibition

The Organic Cation Transporters (OCTs) are the "gates" we've been discussing, which regulate the flow of neurochemicals in the kidneys and in the brain. The gates can be measured, as we've already seen, only if you are taking amino acid supplements. Hinz calls this the "exogenous" (meaning external) state. The "endogenous," or natural, state is when you are not taking any amino acid supplements, and it offers no predictable results from lab tests. If you test in the endogenous (non-supplemented) state, nothing useful can be learned from the testing. I ran many such tests to confirm Dr. Hinz's findings, and, as expected, the results were completely haphazard and useless, a waste of time and money. The reason brain researchers believe you can't accurately measure urinary serotonin and dopamine levels is because prior tests measured urinary levels of people who were in the endogenous state.

Hinz realized that the exogenous state, achieved by taking amino acid supplements, creates "competitive inhibition," meaning that when serotonin and dopamine levels are raised at the same time, they start to fuse together and act as one integrated system. This means that whatever is done to raise serotonin will impact dopamine, and whatever is done to raise dopamine will impact serotonin. By taking dopamine-boosting supplements and opening the dopamine gates, the serotonin gates are also triggered to open, and the levels of both chemicals will change. To mention just one area this impacts, the implications of this explain every known side effect in the treatment of Parkinson's disease, which only boosts up dopamine. It turns out if you supplement with the proper balance of serotonin precursors in people with Parkinson's, the side effects can be avoided. I'll discuss this in detail later in this chapter.

Metabolism, Production, and Transportation of Serotonin and Dopamine

When I was in school studying human physiology, a new world was opened to me to the inner workings of the body and how complex every little thing that happens in our body can be. While you don't have to be a neuroscientist to feel better on an amino acid program, understanding the process may be important to you and help speed along your healing process. Sometimes knowing how something works helps us see a more complete picture. Leonardo Da Vinci conducted dissections studying facial anatomy specifically to be able to paint the Mona Lisa. Knowing the inner-workings of this process may help you achieve your best possible results.

Serotonin and dopamine go through different stages: They are made (or, as scientists say, "synthesized"), they are broken down (or "metabolized"), and they are moved around (called "transportation").

Synthesis of these chemicals occurs only from a collection of specific ingredients: the amino acids 5-HTP and tyrosine, vitamin B6, folate, vitamin C, calcium, and cysteine, a sulfur compound. When you take a single amino acid like 5-HTP, your levels of serotonin increase as enzymes act as catalysts, helping make one chemical from another. An enzyme called "aromatic amino acid decarboxylase" pushes this conversion from 5-HTP over to serotonin. The same enzyme converts tyrosine into dopamine. So as your serotonin production goes up from taking 5-HTP, your dopamine production goes up as well. But if you are not taking tyrosine then forcing the body to make more dopamine will eventually burn up your ability to make dopamine. Your dopamine levels will then drop from taking only the 5-HTP to make more serotonin.

Another of the biochemical steps that occurs as serotonin levels go up from taking 5-HTP involves metabolism. The two enzymes (called COMT and MAO) that break down the additional serotonin you are making also break down dopamine. If you do something to boost serotonin, you increase the breakdown of dopamine, which triggers problems. Taking a single amino acid can improve your symptoms for a little while, but eventually side effects will occur as the opposite neurotransmitter declines.

Transportation works in a similar way. Remember the dual-gate lumen model with the double turnstiles? When you boost serotonin by taking 5-HTP, you open up those gates, or transporters. The odd thing I mentioned earlier happens to be that taking one single amino acid opens the gates for both neurotransmitters. Another one of Hinz's many database-driven revelations proved this. So if you take 5-HTP and serotonin goes up, both gates open, so dopamine rushes into the body through the transporters alongside serotonin. In other words, just upping your serotonin will also flood your system with more dopamine. However, just like with the production issue, if more dopamine rushes into the transporters and you aren't being resupplied with tyrosine to keep your dopamine levels up, eventually dopamine levels will drop.

Sorry for the technical details, but the bottom line is this: If you boost levels of one neurochemical, the production, breakdown, and transport systems in the brain all conspire to lower the opposite brain chemical. This has harsh and severe ramifications for anyone boosting a single brain chemical, and manifests in a horrible way with Parkinson's patients.

Parkinson's Disease

Every physician and, more importantly, every Parkinson's patient knows that once you start on the medications that best treat the disease, you will inevitably start to develop significant side effects, like depression and dyskinesias (painful, distorting involuntary movements of the body). These can become debilitating, causing many people to question the medications' long-term viability, as people are forced to choose between worsening Parkinson's symptoms and the drugs' severe side effects. These negative effects come about as dopamine levels soar from the Parkinson's drug Levadopa, which leads to a depletion of serotonin. These same negative effects can be eliminated with a properly administered amino acid protocol.

I hope many of you reading this remain skeptical and question what I am writing about. Remember I was skeptical myself when I first learned about this work. Much of it seems hard to believe, too good to be true, and if it was even half true then why wouldn't every doctor in the country be ordering these tests for people suffering from depression, anxiety, fatigue, and Parkinson's disease? Don't doctors want to stop this suffering? It's complicated. Non-drug, non-surgical treatments are not taken seriously in the U.S. This has become such a warped medical world that it's against the law to even talk about successful treatments that don't involve drugs or surgery. This solution, however effective and science based it may be, does not fit with the current mind-set of drugs and surgery as the only solutions for all health problems. One great thing about our country is that we are free to choose, and you can choose this program as an option if it proves to make sense to you.

8

. . . .

THE THREE
MAJOR TYPES OF
BRAIN PROBLEMS

There are three different types of brain-related problems. Type 1 is the Deficiency Type, where a necessary component (for example, a nutrient or hormone) is missing or at an inadequate level. Type 2 is the Neuron Bundle Damage Type, where some physical or chemical damage has occurred to the brain. Type 3 is the Genetic Type, and comprises those of us born with neurotransmitter problems, or, as my good friend Lynn says, people who are "swimming in the shallow end of the gene pool." Let me share with you some patient histories so we can gain a clear understanding of these different types of brain disorders.

Type 1: Deficiency Types

Amanda, age 41, was depressed and had been overweight most of her life. When she was a slender eight-year-old, her older sister, who was overweight, goaded Amanda into joining her in her constant overeating. Amanda gained a lot of weight, which she still struggles with today. Up to the time she came to see me she had managed to skate by while living on a diet of junk food and lots of sweets. Amanda was deficient in the amino acids the brain uses to make neurotransmitters because she didn't eat much protein (our sole source of amino acids), and her digestive system was ravaged with a yeast (fungal) overgrowth from all the sugar she consumed (which reduced her ability to absorb nutrients).

Amanda stands as a perfect example of what I call a "Deficiency Type," meaning her brain chemistry problems resulted directly from a deficiency of nutrients. Fixing her brain required two steps. First, she had to give up most of the sweets, which eliminated the fungal overgrowth in her digestive tract. Second, she had to include healthy foods in her diet in order to flood her system with the nutrients she was missing (including amino acids, vitamins, and minerals) and boost her neurotransmitter levels. Amanda, like most Deficiency Types, was able to get her brain in order relatively quickly, and within a few months her depression cleared up as her serotonin and dopamine reached normal levels. Her food cravings also disappeared. Most food cravings go away completely when your brain gets the neurotransmitters it needs.

Type 2: Neuron Bundle Damage Types

Terry and her husband bought older homes and fixed them up. This meant living much of the time in the houses they were remodeling, and this caused Terry to be exposed, year after year, to an extremely high level of chemical toxins, from paint thinners to off-gassing carpet glues. Unlike a contractor who might be exposed to these chemicals during the work day and then go home to a relatively chemical-free house, Terry was surrounded by neurotoxic chemicals day and night. Eventually her system crashed, and she started to develop neurological symptoms, like tremors. Her hands shook so much she couldn't take a photograph without it being blurry, and weakness in her arms and legs made her physically demanding work very difficult.

Terry needed large amounts of supplementation and a long series of lab tests to get her program set up, but the resulting difference in how she felt was well worth the efforts. She also needed to undergo an extensive bout of chemical detoxification. Getting the chemicals and heavy metals stored in her body flushed out took a big strain off her nerve cells and stopped the ongoing damage. She suffered through a lot in her treatment plan, as getting neurotoxins out of the body can sometimes make people feel quite badly. But getting her energy back, being able to drink a cup of coffee without spilling it, and having her extreme fatigue vanish made all the difference in the world to her.

Type 3: Genetic Types

Claire was nine years old when I first started working with her. She would throw tantrums in the mornings, hitting and screaming so severely that many days of the month her parents couldn't get her to go to school. She was obsessive about little things, like needing to have every pencil on her desk lined up exactly in a row, or have her breakfast be perfectly arranged on the plate. If her eggs touched her hash browns, she would run up to her room in a rage. She couldn't focus on school work. We worked together for a year and her behavior improved dramatically. Then we started having set backs, and she had "bad" weeks where her old problems came back just as horrible as before.

Claire finally stabilized, and in the second year of treatment was functioning like a normal kid with normal reactions to the challenges of getting to school and fitting in. Once she reached this point, Claire's mom, Sandy, decided to get tested. She'd had problems controlling her emotions and could go from a zero to a ten in seconds, letting insignificant little things unleash bursts of anger. Sandy also had joint pain and stiffness that was burdensome. Her moods were unstable and all over the map. To top it all off, Claire's grandmother, Florence, age 61, also came in to be tested, as she'd been severely depressed her entire life.

To be honest, I'm a little spaced out at work sometimes. I get really busy with patients, and it's hard for me to remember every little detail about every person. Some of this comes from being overly busy, and some of it is I just don't have the best attention to detail; I get more involved in the people I'm communicating with and sometimes miss out on seeing every lab detail. Sandy one day pointed out to me that her daughter's lab results and her mother's lab results were identical. My first reaction was that wasn't possible; no two people could have the exact same test results. It would be like two people showing up at a party wearing the exact same shirt, pants, shoes, and socks. Possible, but highly unlikely. It turned out that Sandy was absolutely right. In fact, everyone in her family ended up having extremely similar lab results, and although we don't have enough data yet to know for sure, there is clearly a genetic component to some of this.

Type 1: Deficiency Types Explained

If you have one of the common brain problems, including depression, fatigue, anxiety, food cravings, addiction issues, and migraines, you may be a Deficiency Type. This means you don't have enough neurotransmitters, and you need to rebuild or replenish your "empty glass." Once you fill it back up, the problem ends. This might seem too good to be true, but I see it every week as I work with people struggling with these issues. This is the basis of many of the "Dr. Dan, the Miracle Man" stories floating around my clinic, because it seems like a miracle when all of a sudden a person's brain reengages after years of struggling to function without enough serotonin and dopamine to make things work right.

There are many reasons you could be a Deficiency Type, but four main patterns show up most of the time in the people I work with:

1. You can deplete your brain chemicals by burning through them too quickly. This occurs when you are under a lot of stress, don't get enough sleep, etc. I wish we all had some type of meter on our foreheads so everyone could track the amount of stress-related burnout we go through. You literally use up chemicals in your brain as you worry, have fears, get angry, get sad, etc. If someone was sitting next to you, calm and peaceful, their "burn rate" of brain chemicals would be much lower than yours.

2. You can also deplete your brain chemicals by not resupplying your system with the key nutrients needed to make adequate amounts of brain chemicals. All the amino acids and vitamins I've mentioned before don't just appear from out of nowhere; you have to eat foods that supply these nutrients in order to acquire the raw ingredients needed to make brain chemicals. Mostly this means protein, and how many of you eat super healthy protein every day? It's hard to even find super healthy protein, like grass-fed meat, in most grocery stores.

3. Poor digestive function results in poor absorption of nutrients. This can be caused by a lack of digestive enzymes, or by stomach infections from common bad bacterias, such as *H. pylori*. Even if you have a pristine diet, it's possible your digestive system isn't able to absorb all the nutrients your body and brain need.

4. Something that's extremely ironic and tragic is that taking medications like antidepressants lowers brain chemicals over time. This drug-induced depletion has become a bigger problem each year as doctors

continue to overprescribe these medications, and you can't address it by prescribing another drug; you have to test, and fix the deficiency to make up for the side effects of the medications.

Type 2: Neuron Bundle Types Explained

We've detailed this area already, but it bears repeating because this may well be happening to you to some degree without your being aware of the source of the problem. Neurotoxins (the chemicals that destroy nerve cells) and physical injuries cause neuron bundle damage. I recently heard a news report on the radio about three major research studies just completed showing the long-term harm exerted on people from exposure to chemicals. The worst of the three cited a study on babies in utero. It turns out that the more chemicals babies are exposed to in the womb, the higher the chance they will eventually experience mental health problems, from depression to addiction.

I see a similar "new" awareness coming into the world regarding head injuries too. Many news reports come out each month about athletes, from football players to hockey players, that have experienced significant head trauma who are suffering from increased rates of depression, suicide, and other mental health crises. The same story is playing out with veterans returning from Iraq and Afghanistan, where head injuries have become the signature wound.

Regardless of how your brain cells become damaged, in order to restore normal brain functions we must use amino acids to increase your level of neurotransmitters. We will ultimately reach the point where the cells that aren't damaged fire frequently enough to make up for those cells that are unable to fire at all.

Type 3: Genetic Types Explained

Some of us have the bad luck to be born with a genetic tendency for brain problems. If you ask around or think for a while about your own friends and family, you may realize how common this phenomena really is. For instance, every generation of my family has several people with brain problems, including bipolar disorder, major depression, and epilepsy. My best friend's family has a long track record of eating disorders; another friend has two alcoholic parents. It's all around us, really: depression, addiction, eating problems, Parkinson's, Alzheimer's, ADD, autism. I think every family of every person I know has as least one person suffering from a brain problem.

The stories I hear at work about generation after generation of families suffering from addiction and depression, ADD and autism, and all other mental-health related disorders make me irresolute in my determination to help all those I can.

PARKINSON'S DISEASE

Parkinson's disease is the prototype model for the damaged neuron bundle type. In Parkinson's, significant portions of the dopamine-related part of the brain become damaged, resulting in dramatic symptoms as neurons fail to fire properly. This often occurs from exposure to chemicals or heavy metals that act as neurotoxins and destroy delicate brain tissue. Through the careful study of hundreds of Parkinson's cases, Dr. Hinz's database has demonstrated that those with Parkinson's require extraordinary amounts of tyrosine and *Mucuna pruriens* extracts to raise their dopamine to a therapeutic level, but it can be accomplished. And perhaps even more importantly, if dopamine remains the sole focus of a program, Dr. Hinz has shown that serotonin levels will drop.

This single concept, that dopamine and serotonin operate as a system and must be attended to accordingly, is unknown in the Parkinson's research community. What we have found through years of testing is that the acceleration of dopamine levels actually depletes serotonin, and that this serotonin depletion creates most if not all of the vicious side effects of Parkinson's medications.

If you increase dopamine and leave serotonin unattended, you will deplete serotonin by three different mechanisms. It's a bit technical but is worth understanding, especially if you have Parkinson's or if you take any single amino acid. Increasing dopamine increases the enzymes that break down dopamine. These same enzymes also break down serotonin, so serotonin levels drop. Similarly, increasing dopamine increases the enzymes that help you make dopamine, and these same enzymes also help you make serotonin, causing serotonin production to increase. However, without adding 5-HTP to balance things out, this accelerated boost of serotonin leads to a crash. Finally, when dopamine is increased, the gates that both serotonin and dopamine pass through are opened, which further depletes serotonin.

Ultimately, if you take a single amino acid like tyrosine or 5-HTP, you will deplete the opposite neurotransmitter. If you take Parkinson's medications, which increase dopamine, you will experience a significant drop in serotonin, and the classic symptoms will ensue. Lab testing for neurotransmitters solves these potential problems. The combination of being able to exactly calibrate dopamine levels with a lab test and being able to address the inevitable depletion of serotonin from treating Parkinson's with dopamine boosters makes the Hinz protocols a must for any Parkinson's patient at any stage of the disease as an adjunct to help patients tolerate the medications they require.

ADD

For kids and adults alike, Attention Deficit Disorder (ADD) or Attention Deficit Hyperactivity Disorder (ADHD) can be debilitating. Lack of focus and concentration, constantly jumping from thought to thought, can make school or work daunting. Both of these conditions can benefit from the right balance of amino acids. I get to watch this play out in my practice every week; it's a miracle each time, yet as predictable as filling up a gas tank. If you have the proper balance of dopamine and serotonin and everything is "topped off," you'll have a fully functional brain that can think and process, and study and work, without being constantly off track and distracted.

If you have been on medications for these conditions in the past then the amino acid programs can rebuild your levels of missing chemicals regardless of how long you've taken medications like Adderall or Ritalin. I have seen close to 100% success rates treating people with these specific conditions using amino acids. Not to jinx anything, but the brain seems to bounce back quickly with the right program. Most folks I've done this with can taper off their supplement programs and stop all their pills once proper firing in the brain has been reestablished for six to twelve months.

WEIGHT, CRAVINGS, AND ADDICTION

Weight Gain

Did you see the movie *Outbreak* with Morgan Freeman and Dustin Hoffman, or the more recent movie *Contagion*? These types of "viral plague" movies always feature a crash team of experts flying out in the middle of the night from The Centers for Disease Control in Atlanta to save the American population with a last minute vaccination that one of them literally dies to create. Well, in real life the Centers for Disease Control tracks less Hollywood glam things, like how fat our country is getting. Take a minute and go online and check out this link from our nation's premier protector of public health: http://www.cdc.gov/obesity/data/trends.html.

Exactly like the viral plague projections in Outbreak, you can see the plague of obesity spreading throughout the U.S. on the CDC website. Pay special attention to the beginning of the display when the country was all white and light blue, representing 10% or less obesity rates, and then notice how the CDC had to create new colors to track the rising obesity rates in 1997 (beige meaning 20% obesity) and again in 2001 (orange, at 25%). By 2005 a statistician at the CDC clearly became alarmed because they used the color red for the first time, as they now had states with shockingly high 30% obesity rates. What color can they go to next if this trend continues to escalate? All the warning signal systems I've ever seen, such as our homeland security codes, or wild fire danger charts, end at red: maximum overload.

And this display only shows part of the problem. If you take someone my size, at 5'8" and 160 pounds, I'm considered "normal weight." At my height, if I was 165 pounds or over I'd be considered "overweight," but I wouldn't reach the obese category until I hit over 200 pounds! That means if I gained

35 pounds tomorrow, I'd still not be captured by the obesity charts you just looked at. So to make matters even worse, you have to add to the obesity problem another 30% of the population that has become overweight but hasn't yet reached the clinical definition of being obese.

Being trained in clinical nutrition, I clearly see the impact of a poor diet on the increasing obesity rate. However, there is something else even more insidious going on, and it can be challenging to identify. Not only have our diets been stripped of the levels of nutrients we require to function properly, but as I've said over and over, our exposure to environmental toxins has contributed to these growing trends. No amount of medicine can resolve this problem; in fact, dumping more medicinal chemicals into your body in an effort to "fix things" can, in many cases, make this brain drain even worse.

Cravings

See if any of this hits home: Overweight? Food cravings? Have you struggled with binge eating, starving yourself, and dieting? Do you have to have something sweet at night even though you know you shouldn't be hungry? While a lot of you might suffer from the "sugar blues" or blood sugar-related problems that lead to overeating and weight gain, you could also be reacting to low neurotransmitter levels. If you are like me when I was in my 20s and you eat a large bowl of ice cream every night because your serotonin is low, you will eventually develop a blood sugar-handling problem. Trust me when I say that if you exercise enough you can get away with eating extra calories without gaining weight, but that doesn't mean there isn't a serious health problem developing of which you are unaware. A healthy brain means you will have a normal appetite. A normal appetite means that you get hungry if you don't eat for five or six hours, and then after a moderate-sized meal you'll be full, not craving sweets or wanting to overeat. Believe it or not, people with healthy brains eat a small meal and feel full and satisfied and are energized by their food. They tackle the day's activities with a clear mind, with no thoughts about food for another four to six hours or longer.

A drained brain causes your appetite to increase, generating an excessive appetite which then becomes impossible to turn off. You'll be hungry constantly, sometimes even right after a meal. This usually worsens in the late afternoon and evening. The natural low point of neurotransmitter production occurs at 4 p.m., and many people feel this dip in energy and deal with it by consuming sweets. An increase in melatonin production at bedtime that prepares us for sleep can create a significant drop in serotonin, which will trigger food cravings. Think 10 or 11 p.m.—chocolate, ice cream, a bowl of cereal, a handful (or more) of cookies; does this sound familiar? I myself spent many nights cradling a bowl of ice cream before I understood this was my attempt to get my brain chemicals back in balance.

It is easy to overeat at these times in an attempt to gain some temporary relief from the unpleasant feelings generated by this drop in brain chemicals. In fact, some people I've worked with go to extremes and are literally hungry all day long, or find themselves waking up at night to eat, unable to fall back asleep until their cravings have been reduced by overeating on late-night snacks. One significant problem is that this eating behavior only temporarily reduces the cravings, and people are sure to repeat the cycle the next day. This routine of overeating based on poor brain health has become remarkably common in our culture—just think about the CDC charts. It really does represent a spreading epidemic.

Food Addiction

If your food-related problems get out of control, you could easily develop an eating disorder or become a "food addict." More than just overeating occasionally, food addiction means your problem with food has gotten so out of control that you may need professional help to get your diet back on track. By that I mean more than just a few sessions with a nutritionist to learn what the healthy eating habits you need to follow are; you might need the support of counseling or even a twelve step program to get back on track. Addiction to food can become a physical, emotional, and even spiritual problem, and must be addressed on all levels for your recovery.

My personal hero in this work is therapist Lynn Elliott-Harding, who taught me everything I know about food addiction. In my first few years of practice I did notice that some people simply couldn't make the diet changes I suggested; they tried, but couldn't stop eating sugar, or wheat, or simply stop overeating. I really didn't understand what was going on until I met Lynn and began to study the area of addiction.

It turns out that your brain controls your appetite, and if you don't have the right amount of serotonin or dopamine, you are going to try to eat your way out of the problem. Carbs and sweets will give you a short-term boost of brain chemicals and make you feel good for a few hours, but later in the day or the next day the cravings will return and you'll repeat the same overeating patterns again and again.

The total end of cravings for food and the end of overeating is one of the first early effects of balancing your brain chemicals. And it doesn't get just a little better—the cravings stop completely as soon as your serotonin and dopamine levels are balanced.

Alcohol Addiction

Around 14 million people in the US have a problem with alcohol. This means that half of all the adults in this country have a close family member with the problem, and about 25% of children deal with an adult with alcohol issues. Although this problem is all around us, we tend to ignore it. Alcoholism is caused by a variety of reasons, many of which are physiologically or biochemically based, not character or personality based. Some people drink alcohol to buffer low brain chemical problems, just like some of us use food for the same reasons. Some alcoholics make high levels of certain brain chemicals when they drink alcohol. These brain chemicals, or THIQ compounds, hit the system just like an opiate drug such as heroin does, and the alcohol addiction comes about from the brain chemicals produced, not from the alcohol itself. Yet another type of alcoholism comes from blood sugar instability. Some people have EFA-related alcohol cravings. They don't produce chemicals called prostaglandins properly, so when these folks drink alcohol they feel better because their prostaglandin levels go up and they experience a sense of relief, almost a high, just from this shift.

If you have food or alcohol addiction issues, all these variables need to be assessed along with the three key body systems. If you can balance all three body systems and straighten out your brain chemicals, most alcohol cravings will clear up, and abstinence will be much easier to achieve. The struggle people face trying to not drink alcohol or not overeat can be greatly reduced by balancing the brain.

Fatigue: Physical exhaustion that won't leave regardless of rest

Low dopamine manifests as low energy. The lower your dopamine levels, the more exhausted you become. A deep, physical and mental state of fatigue takes over, motivation goes out the window, and the ability to engage in daily activities disappears. The "blahs" set in. Everything seems overwhelming as depression settles over. Low dopamine states do not seem to be accompanied by sadness or regret—more of a worn out feeling that makes it hard for people to pick themselves up and get things done. Lack of rest and the inability to relax and get a good night's sleep further exacerbate the tiredness associated with low dopamine states.

Sleep

Low-serotonin states lead to difficulties sleeping. People struggle with being able to relax and fall asleep at night. This lack of rest compounds the fatigue from the low dopamine and people end up physically spent. In reality it is a bit more complex than this since dopamine and serotonin exist in a balanced state when we are healthy. In fact, it is the balance of serotonin and dopamine that make for a healthy sleep cycle and feelings of energy and well being. It's not a case of a single neurotransmitter causing a single problem.

Food addiction/alcohol addiction, cravings for sugar or alcohol

In a healthy brain, remember, a neuron releases serotonin or dopamine, and these chemicals cause neighboring nerve cells to fire and release an electrical signal, much like a match ignites from a spark. This process then sends messages to the next brain cell. When we obsess on a thought, worrying over and over about something, when we become anxious, or when we crave food or alcohol, it signals that our brain cells are not firing properly.

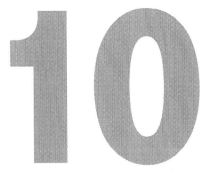

10

GET SMART:
THE HEALTHY
BRAIN LIFESTYLE

We all know how important it is to take good care of our bodies, to eat right, exercise properly, and get adequate sleep. But what about the brain? Most people don't think about "brain care," and just assume the brain will take care of itself. When we do decide to improve our health, most of us turn to exercise, and concentrate solely on growing muscle, or losing fat. Very few people know they should be taking special care of their brains. I doubt even most doctors think about this issue or that they would know what to recommend for basic brain care if you asked.

Basic brain health comes about from taking in the right nutrients so your brain has the fuel it needs to work at full capacity, flushing out stored-up chemicals in the body that damage the brain, and reducing the chemicals you are exposed to that could damage brain cells in the future. In addition to these three specific brain-healing concepts, you can also heal your brain with other general lifestyle changes, including sleep, exercise, and stress management techniques. This chapter will review these areas and give you specific action steps to start your own brain-health program right away.

The Brain-Healthy Diet

You have to eat every day, so you might as well eat to maintain a healthy brain. To start with, be on the lookout for commonly eaten foods that inflame the brain. We are all familiar with inflammation; if you whack your thumb with a hammer, it's inflammation that causes your thumb to swell. Most people, however, aren't aware of inflammation that can exist on the inside of their skulls. Just like any other trauma, foods that trigger inflammation and cause brain swelling will damage brain cells and cause a variety of symptoms, including fatigue, "brain fog," focus and concentration problems, anxiety, and sometimes even depression.

A brain-healthy diet reduces inflammation by avoiding foods that provoke this type of "flame on" response. Food choices center around an organic, whole-foods diet with plenty of high-quality organic protein, good fats, and no refined foods or artificial sugars. In short, it is a chemical-free diet that is more in alignment with the diet your great-grandparents probably ate. By following this type of diet, you will feel better physically, have more energy, eliminate cravings, improve sleep quality, and probably lose weight. To attain your optimum brain health through diet, it is helpful to eliminate gluten, soy, and pasteurized dairy for at least two months. This will reduce inflammation in your brain and help it repair, and at the same time focus on maintaining stable blood sugar to keep your cravings under control.

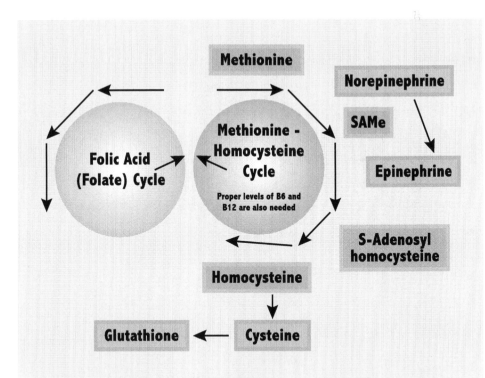

In order to make neurotransmitters, we need a large supply of nutrients that are often lacking in the modern American diet.

FOODS ALLOWED

Proteins

Protein is the framework of the brain-healthy diet, because protein breaks down into the amino acids that are the precursors to the production of your feel-good neurotransmitters. High-quality protein sources include grass-fed beef, bison, and lamb; free-range poultry and free-range eggs; wild fish; and organic, farm-raised pork. It is very important that you eat adequate protein—around four ounces, or a piece about the size of your palm—at each meal. The variety of protein sources and quality are of utmost importance. Protein should be organic, hormone-free, free-range, grass-fed, and "wild caught" in the case of fish. Conventional, factory-farmed meat is full of brain toxins, nasty hormones, and antibiotics that will muddle your brain function.

Use only fresh meats; avoid those that are processed and packaged. It is important to divide your day's total protein over the course of your day. An easy starting point for calculating the amount of protein you need is to divide your ideal body weight (in pounds) by 15 to get the ounces of protein to be consumed per day. You will need to adjust this amount up or down depending on your genetic type, the health of your metabolism, and your activity level.

Beef, pork, and lamb: local if possible, and always grass fed. Grain-fed cattle have altered fatty acid ratios that increase inflammatory components in the beef and inflame your brain.

Fish: Eat a variety of grilled, steamed, baked, or poached, but do not bread or deep-fry. Do not consume canned tuna due to its mercury levels. Choose "wild-caught" fish and avoid larger fish such as shark, mackerel, and tuna due to their high mercury contents.

Poultry: Eat a variety of chicken, turkey, and game hen, in a mix of dark and white meat. Do not bread or deep-fry. Acceptable cooking methods are grilled, steamed, baked, or roasted.

Eggs: The yolk has nutrients that are denatured when cooked thoroughly, so eat your eggs soft-boiled, sunny side up, or over-easy when you can. Buy organic eggs from a local farmer if possible, and notice their bright orange yolks! This equates to high levels of brain-healthy omega-3 fatty acids.

Nuts: These may be used as a protein snack source. Raw and organic are preferable. You can also soak nuts for easy digestibility.

Cheese: Goat and sheep cheeses and goat or sheep milk yogurt are great alternatives to cow dairy products, which should be avoided until dairy sensitivity is ruled out.

Carbohydrates

Unrefined carbohydrates include vegetables, fruits, grains, and beans. Refined carbohydrates are man-made processed foods that may contain white flour, white sugar, corn, or corn syrup. Unrefined carbs feed your brain, while refined carbs cause problems. Refined carbs have been processed and stripped of their essential nutrients, and will throw off your insulin levels, cause inflammation, and wreak general havoc with your brain health. In stark contrast, unrefined carbs are rich in vitamins and minerals and will feed your brain what it needs to operate properly. I know your mother told you this a thousand times, but she was right: Eat your vegetables.

Vegetables

Nutrient-rich vegetables provide the vitamins and minerals that sustain your body. Again, quality and variety are key. Your body is most nourished with high-quality organic produce. Many anti-inflammatory, brain-healing nutrients such as antioxidants and flavinoids are associated with the properties that give vegetables their color, so make sure you eat a good range of green, yellow, red, and even purple veggies. Eating vegetables raw or lightly cooked helps maintain vitamin and mineral content.

Green vegetables: Eat as many of these as you can. They are high in minerals and low in calories. Some examples include swiss chard, kale, collard greens, bok choy, beet greens, spinach, and salad greens. Dark-green steamed vegetables are superior to salad greens.

Yellow and orange vegetables: Eat these in small portions and always balance with green vegetables and protein. Some examples include yams, winter squash, and carrots.

Onions & garlic: Eat these as desired. They provide a good source of sulfur-containing amino acids that enhance liver detox function and protect your brain cells from neurotoxins.

Fruits

Whole fresh seasonal fruits are good in moderation. Best picks include berries, citrus, melons, apples, and pears. Avoid dried fruit, which is very high in sugar and may contain harmful preservatives.

Grains

Gluten-free grains are best (if you choose to consume grains at all), including amaranth, arrowroot, buckwheat, corn, millet, quinoa, and white or brown rice. There are now rice breads and millet breads available for toast and sandwiches, as well as rice, corn, and quinoa-based pastas. So you can still eat the regular foods you are used to while keeping your diet gluten-free.

Legumes

Legumes such as beans and lentils are an excellent source of carbohydrates.

Fats

If protein is the framework to a brain-healthy diet, then fats are the nails and the bolts. The brain is 80 percent fat, so it is crucial to have unrefined fat sources at each meal. Fat also increases absorption of the fat-soluble vitamins A, D, E, and K. As with all food groups, it is important to give your body a variety. Choose from extra-virgin cold-pressed olive oil, sesame oil, cod liver oil, virgin unrefined coconut oil, and real butter or ghee. Raw butter is ideal because it possesses healing qualities. Avoid all margarines and hydrogenated and partially hydrogenated oils, as well as canola oil and other vegetable oils. Butter and coconut oil are the most stable when heating or stir-frying. Always buy organic, cold-pressed oils in glass containers, not plastic.

Brain cells can only function when properly supplied with sufficient omega-3 fats, most often found in fish. Because it's hard to get enough of these fats from your diet alone these days, most people need to supplement with a good quality omega fish oil supplement.

Beverages

Water is the best beverage to drink. Our bodies are 70 percent water, and water is considered a nutrient, optimizing digestive function and the elimination of toxins from your body. It's best to avoid too much caffeine, fruit juices, and alcoholic beverages, especially beer, which contains gluten. If you are a daily caffeine consumer, don't quit right away. Start by making improvements in your diet and exercise patterns, and your need for the extra boost that caffeine provides will fade over time. Coffee is very acidic to the body, which accelerates the aging process.

FOODS TO AVOID

Gluten

Although not everyone is gluten intolerant, everyone stands to benefit from a gluten-free diet for two months. It forces us to eat less of the processed, refined foods that contain gluten, and eat more unprocessed foods such as organic vegetables, quality proteins, fats, and healthy carbohydrates. Starchy foods that are allowed include amaranth, arrowroot, buckwheat, corn, millet, potato, quinoa, and rice. Oats are tolerated by most gluten-sensitive people, but are controversial as to their actual gliadin content, so always be a little suspicious about oats; if you get bloated after eating oatmeal or granola, then remove them from your diet.

Soy

Soy consumption has become quite controversial. Once considered a magic bullet, soy was thought to offer cardio-protective properties, cancer prevention, and menopause relief. We now know that soy consumption is linked to hormonal cancers, thyroid issues, impaired fertility, food allergies, and infant abnormalities.

The majority of soy produced in the U.S. has been genetically modified. Genetic modification provides resistance to toxic herbicides, but the result is that soy plants contain genes from bacteria that produce a protein that has never been part of the human food supply. It is still too early for us to know the full repercussions of genetically modified foods in our diet. In addition, soy is very difficult to digest and contains many anti-nutrients that prevent absorption of minerals. Soy also contains high levels of plant estrogens that mimic the body's natural estrogens, and consumption of soy products can cause estrogen dominance in certain individuals. Estrogen dominance raises one's risk of hormonal cancers and female hormone issues.

In our current diets, we very rarely consume whole soy. It is processed into soy flours, soy oil, soy protein isolate, and hydrolyzed soy protein and is ubiquitous in our food supply because it is cheap to produce. It's used in processed foods as filler, and is a main ingredient in vegetarian fare, protein powders, supplements, and protein bars.

Avoid processed soy as much as possible. Many people are allergic to soy and soy products. Part of this may stem from the ways in which soy has been genetically modified, and the frequency with which it is used as a food additive. Fermented soy products such as miso, natto, and tempeh are usually all right. After a long fermentation process, the phytate levels of soybeans are reduced, making them much easier to digest. Because soy allergy is so common, remove it from your diet for at least a month and reintroduce it to see if it causes unpleasant symptoms such as indigestion or bloating.

Pasteurized Dairy

Reactions to pasteurized dairy products are very common, but they may be so subtle that you may not even notice. This includes pasteurized milk, cheese, yogurt, and cottage cheese, but not eggs. There are two potential problems with dairy products: lactose intolerance, which is an inability to digest the carbohydrate or sugar portion of the milk, and milk allergy, which is a reaction to the protein in the milk. Pasteurization and homogenization destroy the enzymes in milk that help us digest it, destroy the healthy bacteria in milk that help keep the gut working well, and destroy the beneficial fats in dairy, rendering what could be a very nurturing and healing food into a potentially harmful product.

Dairy sensitivity may manifest as bloating, diarrhea, sinus and hay fever symptoms, and generalized digestive complaints. While pasteurized dairy should be avoided, raw dairy may be introduced after two weeks of following a dairy-free diet. After two weeks, most people will be able to tell if they are sensitive to dairy by drinking a large glass of whole raw milk first thing in the morning on an empty stomach. If you have no digestive symptoms from doing this, then you can likely consume raw dairy products. Raw butter has butyric acid, which along with the healthy bacteria in the butter helps heal the GI tract in dramatic ways.

RENEW DETOXIFICATION PROGRAM INSTRUCTIONS

There are foods that help you detox and foods that impede the process of cleansing

	Foods That Increase Detoxification	Foods To Avoid
Fruits	Raspberries, Strawberries, Blueberries 100% Berry Juices Bananas, Apples Any other fresh or frozen fruit	Canned fruit packed in syrup High sugar or artificial berry juices Oranges
Vegetables	Broccoli, Cabbage, Cauliflower Brussels Sprouts, Watercress Arugula, Kale, Bok Choy, Radish, Turnip Beans and Lentils Garlic, Onion	Corn Canned vegetables in sauces Soybean and soy-based foods
Grains, etc.	Rice-whole grain Buckwheat Millet Amaranth Quinoa	Refined flours Gluten-containing grains - Wheat - Rye - Spelt - Oats* - Kamut - Barley
Nuts, etc.	Almonds, Cashews, Walnuts Sunflower seeds Sesame seeds	Peanuts Soy nuts
Dairy	None - Use a milk substitute like Rice Milk or Almond Milk	Milk Cheese Ice cream Yogurt All dairy-based products
Fats	Extra virgin olive oil Flaxseed oil Nut oils other than peanut	Margarine Butter Hydrogenated oils
Drinks	Purified Water 100% fruit or vegetable juices Organic Herbal Tea Organic Green Tea	Coffee Sweetened Beverages Alcohol High Sugar or artificially flavored juices Black Tea
Spices/Sauces	Rosemary, Parsley, Cilantro , Thyme	Soy sauce, BBQ sauce, Ketchup
Other		Eggs Fish and Shellfish Non-organic meats Fried Foods Artificial flavors, colors, preservatives (MSG)

* Oats do not contain gluten, however commercially available oats often are contaminated with gluten.
  It is best to avoid oats.

NOTE: Individuals with joint pain should consider avoiding foods derived from the nightshade family of plants
[such as tomatoes, white potatoes, eggplant, peppers of all kinds (except black pepper), paprika, and cayenne]

157

Food Allergies and Rotation Diets

Food allergies are becoming a more widely recognized health problem. Often it is not clear which foods are causing reactions. When I have patients who are experiencing food allergies or sensitivities, I suggest that they get a simple lab test to determine the specific foods they are allergic to, and then go on a rotation diet. For most people, a four-day rotation interval between eating the same foods gives the best results. The food being rotated on a given day may be eaten more than once. Rotation diets are complex to follow and typically require the help of a health professional to do properly.

Once you have a brain-healthy diet sorted out, you can turn your sights to cleaning out the junk that has accumulated in your brain tissue over the years.

Detoxing the Brain: Clogged Detox Pathways

As I mentioned earlier, a couple years ago I left the safety of my California home and ventured to Ohio for a family gathering. As we were leaving the airport in Cleveland in our rental car I started to feel sick, and I quickly realized it was that "new car smell." The off-gassing of the chemicals from that rental car's interior literally made me nauseous, and we had to drive to Akron with the windows down when it was 20 degrees outside! At the hotel I took a shower in the most highly chlorinated water I could imagine, and the next three days were a chemical exposure fest that made me spacey, tired, and a little depressed. I learned that while you can protect yourself at home, it's not so easy to do everywhere, and unless you take extreme measures, you will be exposed to a bewildering number of chemicals, heavy metals, and other poisons in your environment each day. Your body's ability to remove these harmful toxins can easily be overwhelmed, leaving you tired and toxic. Your body has a threshold for the amount of toxins it is able to effectively process and excrete. When this threshold is exceeded due to exposure to household and environmental chemicals, toxins will build up in your body and cause symptoms.

Your liver is your body's hardest working organ, in charge of detoxifying every single thing you breathe, eat, drink, and apply to your skin. Your liver flushes out toxins like a washing machine flushes dirt from your clothes. The liver can become overworked and congested due to caffeine, alcohol, drugs, heavy metals, pesticides, and fumes, as well as chemicals in our food, drinking water, and environment. At that point it is not able to effectively get rid of toxins, and they end up being stored in your fat cells. These accumulated toxins can be removed from the body via sweating, urinating, bowel movements, and breathing, so if any of these processes are compromised (constipation, for example, or if you don't drink enough water), elimination of toxins becomes impaired.

Toxins such as pollution, exhaust, solvents, pesticides, and heavy metals also have the ability to cross the blood-brain barrier, which is designed to keep harmful chemicals away from brain tissue. You may be exposed to these chemicals daily by eating conventionally sprayed produce, breathing outdoors in an urban area, eating fish high in mercury, drinking diet sodas, applying cosmetics like lipstick or lotions to your skin, and from common household cleaners.

Exposure to neurotoxins is a common reason for imbalanced brain chemistry. Remember, neuron bundles are damaged by neurotoxins, and this damage reduces the neuron's ability to fire properly. Children may be especially vulnerable to the health risks of pesticides and other chemicals because of their developing brains. A recent study found disturbingly high levels of pesticide compounds in a staggering 94 percent of children tested. The compounds break down in the body and can be measured in urine. Children with higher levels of chemicals and pesticides have increased chances of having ADHD.

Neurotoxins like pesticides and aluminum can cause chronic neurodegenerative diseases in adults, leading to an increased risk of Parkinson's disease, Alzheimer's disease, and depression. Studies have shown that pesticide exposure increases Parkinson's and other neurodegenerative diseases up to 70 percent because these chemicals destroy the dopamine-related portion of the brain called the *substantia nigra*. On a less dramatic scale, neurotoxins can cause migraines, fibromyalgia-type pain, depression, and insomnia.

Excitotoxins

What about artificial sweeteners versus real sugar? Are you now consuming or have you ever in the past drunk diet sodas or sugar-free drinks sweetened with aspartame or saccharine? These fake sugar substitutes are neurotoxins known as "excitotoxins" which cross the blood-brain barrier and cause brain cell death. Fake sugars are linked to headaches and migraines, dizziness, seizures, nausea, numbness, muscle spasms, rashes, depression, fatigue, irritability, tachycardia, insomnia, vision problems, hearing loss, heart palpitations, breathing difficulties, anxiety attacks, slurred speech, loss of taste, tinnitus, vertigo, memory loss, and joint pain.

Did you know that aspartame and other fake sugars are also linked to weight gain? Studies suggest that aspartame may actually stimulate appetite and bring on a craving for carbohydrates. Researchers believe that tasting any kind of sweet taste will signal an insulin release, which causes the body to store carbohydrates and fats. This can, in turn, cause the body to crave more food. In an article in the San Francisco Chronicle, writer Jean Weininger states that, "Studies have shown that people who use artificial sweeteners don't necessarily reduce their consumption of sugar—or their total calorie intake." Finally, the American Cancer Society (1986) documented the fact that persons using artificial sweeteners gain more weight than those who avoid them.

Aspartame has been controversial since its approval as a food additive by the U.S. Food and Drug Administration (FDA) in 1981. Although countless studies have proven otherwise, the FDA maintains that aspartame is a safe food additive. It is marketed under the names Equal and NutraSweet and is found in over 6,000 foods and drinks. Aside from diet sodas, aspartame is also found in mints, gum, candy, sugar-free desserts, yogurt, ketchup, and nutrition bars. Do your brain, your weight, and your overall health a favor and cut out the diet sodas and fake sugar substitutes.

MSG, or monosodium glutamate, is another excitotoxin to watch out for. Some people experience reactions after eating MSG. These reactions include migraine headaches, upset stomach, fuzzy thinking, diarrhea, heart irregularities, asthma, and mood swings. MSG is disguised under many aliases, including autolyzed yeast, hydrolyzed protein, textured protein, calcium caseinate, sodium caseinate, and maltodextrin. It is also hidden in many stocks, bouillons, or broths; any "flavors" or "flavorings"; and many seasonings. By avoiding processed foods, you'll avoid MSG.

Clean, Clear Water

Now that you've given up your processed junk food and diet soda, you'll be drinking more water. But don't fill up your plastic bottle with tap water. Get rid of the plastic, which leaches chemicals into your drinking water, and replace it with a stainless steel water canteen or, better yet, a glass one. And regardless of what you've heard about the quality of your city's tap water, avoid water from the tap whenever possible.

Most municipal water flows through older lead pipes that contain toxins and pollutants, both before reaching the water treatment plant and also afterwards on its way to your house. Some chemicals that have been found in tap water include the following: perchlorate, a compound found in rocket fuel; arsenic, mercury, and other neurotoxic heavy metals; herbicides and pesticides; hormones such as estrogen; and hexavalent chromium, a cancer-causing chemical. If this isn't enough to convince you, the chlorine that is used to disinfect our water combines easily with other chemicals and naturally occurring organic materials to form other carcinogenic substances. An example of one of these resulting carcinogens is trihalomethane, a chemical which is not only associated with cancer but also with nervous system damage. Consider installing a water filtration system, such as one that attaches directly to your faucet head.

Mercury

If tap water isn't enough, another major source of heavy metals can be found right in your mouth—in the form of mercury fillings or amalgams.

Mercury is extremely neurotoxic and has a particular affinity for brain tissue. Aside from uranium, mercury is the most toxic metal known to man; it takes only a few milligrams to kill you, and once it accumulates in your tissues, it not only causes neurological problems, but also organ damage. Mercury toxicity in humans has been linked to chronic fatigue syndrome, cardiovascular disease, and kidney problems, and some believe it's contributing to the alarming rise in autism and Alzheimer's disease.

Mercury compounds can enter the body through various pathways, including inhalation of its vapor, ingestion, and skin contact. It's found in paints, pesticides, batteries, fluorescent light bulbs, skin creams, vaccines, old-style thermometers, eye drops, and, of course, those silver amalgam fillings in your mouth. Despite the American Dental Association's best efforts to downplay the risk, mercury from amalgams is continually released, increasing as you chew food or gum. Experts believe that up to 80 percent of mercury released from fillings is retained by the body.

After ingestion, mercury binds with proteins and amino acids and is transported freely throughout the body, accumulating in tissues and crossing the blood-brain barrier. It is then stored in the brain, wreaking havoc on the central nervous system. Over time, mercury leads to oxidative damage, mitochondrial dysfunction, and eventually cell death.

In regards to limiting mercury exposure, pay attention to your living environment. Use chemical-free household cleaning agents and cosmetics. Limit high-risk fish consumption such as tuna, mackerel, and shark. Hook up home air and water filtration systems. In regards to dental health, over three-quarters of adults have amalgam fillings, which should be removed by a dentist experienced in amalgam removal.

Living a Brain-Healthy Lifestyle

We are an extension of our environment, which is currently unhealthy. We are living in a toxic world that has soaked up years of pollutants and chemicals. Consider this: Every time farmland is sprayed with pesticides, these chemicals soak into the earth and find their way into our groundwater. The runoff makes its way to our oceans, lakes, and rivers, and farm workers who harvest the crops are exposed to neurotoxic chemicals. The cotton that is harvested for our clothes is soaked in pesticides that eventually find their way into the fabric that lies against our skin. Every day we put gas and oil into our cars, and we inhale the toxic fumes that cars emit. We sit in front of a computer that expels EMFs at us for eight hours, eat a lunch of processed foods, then go home and clean our homes with toxic household cleaning products. We're stressed, so we drink a beer to relax and eat a pint of ice cream before bed. It's no wonder we're sick.

We've had a direct hand in the environmental degradation we're seeing, and now we are becoming living extensions of toxic living. The brain diseases I have discussed in this book are all a direct result of toxicity. By making changes to our diets and lifestyle, we can do our part to lighten the toxic load on our bodies—and the earth.

Environment

We make choices every day that impact the health of the environment. Many of us recycle or try to buy locally grown food to reduce fossil fuel costs and contamination. We have become a culture driven by commerce and waste, but this model is not sustainable. Recycling and composting are essential to the health of the planet, and these practices cut down on the pollution in our environment. In turn, we are healthier as a result of breathing cleaner air or eating plants that have been grown in healthy soil. Drinking filtered water, eating organic and preferably local meat and produce, using non-toxic cleaning agents, chemical-free cosmetics, and even wearing organic clothing are all key factors in restoring the health of our planet.

Exercise

Exercise helps take off weight, increases energy, improves circulation, and prevents depression. Exercise is a great source of stress relief and can impact the brain at least as powerfully as any antidepressant medication, and without the negative side effects. You'll do best to combine cardio, strength training, stretching, and relaxation exercises in an integrated program.

A properly designed exercise program will include relaxation exercises if you are stressed, resistance training to strengthen muscle, stretching to resolve muscle tension patterns, and cardiovascular exercise to improve overall fitness. If you are in Stage 3 of adrenal burnout, you may require some time healing your adrenal glands before you are able to undertake heavy cardiovascular exercise.

Emotional and Spiritual Health

Emotional and spiritual well-being has played a primary role in the health of every one of the patients I have treated. Our emotional health revolves around our ability to communicate with others and maintain intimacy with those we love. In our culture, we often don't get the right experiences or training that lead to the development of emotionally intimate relationships. It requires practice and hard work, and sometimes therapy or counseling. Regarding our spiritual lives, some people discover the spiritual part of themselves through organized religion, while others find it through a less formal belief system or practice. Achieving satisfying emotional and spiritual health will directly affect your physical health and well-being. For most of us, this is the most important and challenging step toward optimum health.

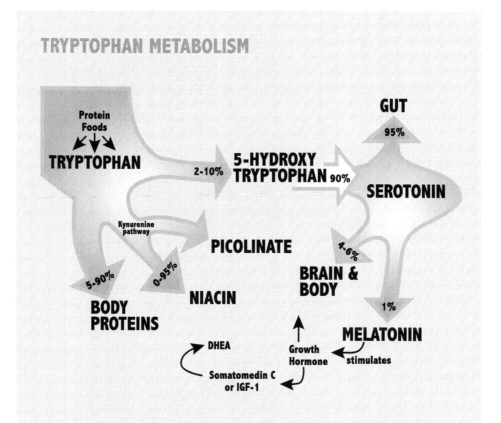

TRYPTOPHAN METABOLISM

The quality of the protein you eat determines the quality and quantity of your brain chemicals.

Reducing Toxin Exposure

Many common sense practices will help you avoid toxin exposure. For example, using "green" household cleaning products, laundry soaps, and beauty products, along with avoiding chemicals and preservatives in your food, all help. Also, installing a shower filter that pulls out chlorine and using fluoride-free toothpaste make a difference. Many excellent books on the subject, including "Supernatural Mom," by Beth Greer, lay out in detail how you can achieve a low-chemical lifestyle.

Sleep

Most of us think of sleep as something to fit in between late night TV shows and getting up to go to work, but we can pay a price for this cavalier attitude. Our brains repair while we sleep. Your brain processes information, detunes itself on a psychic level through dreams and deep sleep cycles, and refreshes our minds for the following day. Both physical repair and psychic regeneration happen at night while we rest. One of the primary means for maintaining a healthy brain is to get a good night's sleep, going to bed around 10 p.m. and waking up when the sun rises.

Stress Management

A million different ways of de-stressing can be used. Some people golf, while others do yoga or garden. We all need to take our minds off of work and the high-stress parts of life so we can refocus and relax. My several years of training in monasteries in Asia gave me excellent stress management skills, and I still meditate regularly as a means of keeping my brain in balance. We each have our own ways of doing this; it's just a matter of making sure that we allow time in our busy lives for relaxing activities.

Nutritional Supplements

A simple 30-day cleanse program done twice yearly can enhance your health and assist in removing neurotoxins that have accumulated in your brain and body. In addition to following the brain-healthy diet, toxins can be removed by using a combination of liver-cleansing herbs and amino acids. Liver cells require nutrients such as taurine, cysteine, glycine, glutamine, choline, and methionine in order to dump out toxins. In addition, a liver-support product that contains antioxidants will counteract any free radicals produced as toxins are pulled from the system. Nutrients that bind to chemicals, toxins, and heavy metals and rid them from the body are essential. Foods that assist the body in accomplishing this include chlorella, cilantro, onions, garlic, cruciferous vegetables, and protein.

The list of brain-healthy nutrients includes cysteine, N-acetyl cysteine (NAC), antioxidants, sulfur compounds, vitamin B6, vitamin C, minerals, selenium, calcium, and folate. You can determine the exact levels you require to have a healthy brain through lab testing, or you can follow a more general program as outlined in the appendix of this book.

APPENDIX

. . . .

These are some of the forms I use in my clinic to help me assess a new patient's overall health. I use these questionnaires as rough guides to point me in the right direction; please don't use them to try to diagnose your own condition. I included them in the appendix so that you might get a better idea of what to expect—what questions might be asked of you—during your initial visit(s) with a functional medicine practitioner trained in The Kalish Method.

BLOOD SUGAR INSTABILITY QUESTIONNAIRE

Name:_____

Yes	No	DO ANY OF THE FOLLOWING APPLY TO YOU?
		Family history of diabetes, hypoglycemia, or alcoholism
		Calmer after meals
		Frequent thirst
		Night sweats (not menopausal)
		Crave salty foods
		Dark circles under eyes or eyes sensitive to bright light
		More awake at night
		Food cravings
		Headaches
		Irritability
		Mood swings
		Easily fatigued
		Anxiety
		Difficulty sleeping
		Mental sluggishness
		Eat when nervous
		Hungry between meals
		Irritable before meals
		"Shaky" if hungry
		Lightheaded if skip meals
		Low energy in afternoon
		Afternoon headaches
		Crave sweets or coffee in afternoon

SOCIAL READJUSTMENT RATING SCALE*

Check YES or NO to each event that has happened to you in the past year. Total up the number of questions answered YES.

LIFE EVENT	YES	NO	POINT VALUE	SCORE
Death of spouse			100	
Divorce			73	
Marital separation			65	
Jail term			63	
Death of close family member			63	
Personal injury or illness			53	
Marriage			50	
Fired from work			47	
Marital reconciliation			45	
Retirement			45	
Change in family member's health			44	
Pregnancy			40	
Sex difficulties			39	
Addition to family			39	
Business readjustment			39	
Change in financial status			38	
Death of close friend			37	
Change in line of work			36	
Change in # of marital arguments			35	
Mortgage or loan over $250,000			31	
Foreclosure of mortgage or loan			30	
Change in work responsibilities			29	
Son or daughter leaving home			29	
Trouble with in-laws			29	
Outstanding personal achievement			28	
Spouse begins or stops work			26	
Starting or finishing school			26	
Change in living conditions			25	

LIFE EVENT	YES	NO	POINT VALUE	SCORE
Revision of personal habits			24	
Trouble with boss			23	
Change in work hours, conditions			20	
Change in residence			20	
Change in schools			20	
Change in recreational habits			19	
Change in church activities			18	
Mortgage or loan under $250,000			18	
Change in sleeping habits			16	
Change in # of family gatherings			15	
Change in eating habits			15	
Vacation			13	
Christmas season			12	
Minor violation of the law			11	

TOTAL SCORE: _____

150 or less:
37% chance of illness within the next two years.

151-299:
50% chance of illness within the next two years.

300 or above:
80% chance of illness within the next two years.

* Holmes, TH and Rahe, RH Booklet for Schedule of Recent Experience (SRE) Seattle, University of Washington, 1967

ADRENAL STRESS PROFILE QUESTIONNAIRE

Next to each question assign a number between 0 and 5. You should assign values as follows:

0 = Not true   3 = Somewhat true   5 = Very true

Once you have completed the questionnaire calculate your total and locate the range you fall under on page two.

	LIFE EVENT
	I experience problems falling asleep.
	I experience problems staying asleep.
	I frequently experience a second wind (high energy) late at night.
	I have energy highs and lows throughout the day.
	I feel tired all the time.
	I need caffeine (coffee, tea, cola, etc) to get going in the morning.
	I usually go to bed after 10 p.m.
	I frequently get less than 8 hours of sleep per night.
	I am easily fatigued.
	Things I used to enjoy seem like a chore lately.
	My sex drive is lower than it used to be.
	I suffer from depression, or have recently been experiencing feelings of depression, such as sadness or loss of motivation.
	If I skip meals I feel low energy or foggy and disoriented.
	My ability to handle stress has decreased.
	I find that I am easily irritated or upset.
	I have had one or more stressful major life events (i.e., divorce, death of a loved one, job loss, new baby, new job).
	I tend to overwork with little time for play or relaxation for extended periods of time.
	I crave sweets.
	I frequently skip meals or eat sporadically.
	I am experiencing increased physical complaints such as muscle aches, headaches, or more frequent illnesses.

SCORING YOUR ADRENAL STRESS PROFILE:

It is important to note that this is not a diagnostic test and should not be used to diagnose any conditions. It is simply a tool to help assess your likely level of adrenal burnout.

If you scored between:

0 – 30   You are in good health.
30 – 40   You are under some stress.
40 – 50   You are a candidate for adrenal burnout.
50 – 60   You are in adrenal burnout.
60 +   You are in severe adrenal burnout.*

* If you scored 60 or higher it is important that you take immediate steps to correct this condition before your health is adversely affected.

If you have scored 40 or higher you are in adrenal burnout and will at some point experience the symptoms such as fatigue, weight gain, insomnia, irritability, and mood swings.

Everyone is under one form of stress or another. A certain amount of stress can be healthy and keep us productive. However, extreme stress can accumulate and start to negatively impact our health, leading to adrenal burnout. Adrenal burnout is all too common in our modern society. Some of the symptoms include: fatigue, weight gain, insomnia, irritability, and mood swings. If you suffer from any of these conditions, take the following questionnaire to identify your personal stress level.

What is Adrenal Burnout?

Your adrenal glands produce your stress hormones, or "adrenaline," the main one being cortisol. Cortisol is released in response to stress. It gives your body a surge of energy to help you respond properly. Stress can come in many forms.

- **Physical stress** - such as an injury or accident.
- **Emotional stress** - such as a demanding career, the birth of a new baby, or the death of a loved one.
- **Environmental stress** - such as pollution, pesticides, or carcinogens.

There are also hidden forms of stress such as inflammation or infections in the gastrointestinal system and food allergies.

Whatever the form of the stress, the adrenal glands are the first to react. If there is a period of prolonged stress, eventually the adrenal glands burn out and are no longer able to produce the amount of cortisol that is required by the body. At this point you may begin to experience symptoms such as fatigue, insomnia, weight gain, irritability, and an inability to cope with stress.

DETOXIFICATION QUESTIONNAIRE

Name:_____ Date:_____

Read the following questions and rate them based on how you have been feeling in the past 30 days.

Fill in the number that applies on the form below:

KEY: 0 (or leave blank) = No or never or almost never occurs
1 = Occasionally occurs, effect is not severe
2 = Occasionally occurs, effect is severe
3 = Frequently occurs, effect is not severe
4 = Frequently occurs, effect is severe

0-4	GASTROINTESTINAL
	Belching or gas
	Heartburn or acid reflux
	Bloating or abdominal discomfort shortly after eating
	Bad breath (halitosis)
	Aggravated by certain foods
	Diarrhea, chronic
	Undigested food in stool
	Constipation
	Nausea or vomiting
	Fewer than one bowel movement a day
	Stools are loose and unformed
_____	**TOTAL**

0-4	LIVER
	Wine makes you sick
	Easily intoxicated if drinking alcohol
	Hangovers after drinking alcohol
	Sensitive to chemicals (perfume, solvents, exhaust)
	Sensitive to tobacco smoke
	Hemorrhoids or varicose veins
	Bothered by aspartame (NutraSweet)
	Chronic fatigue or Fibromyalgia
	Feeling wired or jittery if drinking coffee
	Feet have a strong odor
	Sweat has a strong odor
_____	**TOTAL**

0-4	NAILS
	Ridged nails
	Splitting nails
	White spots on nails
	Crumbling nails
_____	**TOTAL**

0-4	EARS
	Ear infections
	Ear drainage or discharge
	Itchy ears
	Ringing in the ears
_____	**TOTAL**

0-4	SKIN
	Experience hives, cysts, boils, rashes
	Cold sores, fever blisters, or herpes lesions
	Dry flaky skin and/or dandruff
	Fragile skin, easily chafed, as in shaving
	Acne
	Itchy skin / dermatitis
	Dull-colored skin, yellowish, pale or grayish
	Pale complexion
	Skin has a sour or unpleasant odor
_____ TOTAL	

0-4	MOUTH AND THROAT
	Coated tongue (yellow, grayish-white or thick film)
	Swollen tongue
	Hoarseness
	Difficulty swallowing
	Lump in throat
	Dry mouth, eyes, and/or nose
	Gag easily or need to clear throat often
	Mouth ulcers or canker sores
_____ TOTAL	

0-4	EYES
	Dark circles around the eyes
	Puffy eyelids
	Bags under the eyes
	Bloodshot or reddened eyes
	Whites of eyes are yellowed
	Inflamed eyelids
	Eyes are watery and/or itchy
	Blurred or tunnel vision
_____ TOTAL	

0-4	HEART/LUNGS
	Asthma
	Wheezing or difficulty breathing
	Shortness of breath
	Chest congestion
	Heart races, rapid heartbeat
	Fast pulse at rest
	Flush or blush easily, or face turns red for no reason
	Heart skips beats
_____ TOTAL	

0-4	HEAD
	Tension headaches at base of skull
	Splitting-type headache
	Dizziness
	Faintness
_____ TOTAL	

0-4	MENTAL EMOTIONAL
	Feel spacey, thinking seems slow or fuzzy
	Bizarre, vivid, or nightmarish dreams
	Depressed
	Worried, apprehensive, anxious
	Nervous or agitated
	Mentally sluggish, reduced initiative
	Difficulty concentrating
	Mood swings
	Coordination is poor
	Poor memory
_____ TOTAL	

0-4	METABOLISM
	Pulse speeds after eating
	Night sweats
	MSG sensitivity
	Mood swings associated with periods (PMS)
	Breast tenderness associated with cycle
_____ TOTAL	

0-4	WEIGHT
	Crave bread or noodles
	Crave certain foods
	Retaining water
	Excessive weight
_____ TOTAL	

0-4	MUSCULOSKELETAL
	Pain or swelling in joints
	Muscles become easily fatigued
	Muscle aches and pains
	Arthritic tendencies
	Joints are painful upon waking
	Joint pain after mild exertion
	Joint pain experienced after eating certain foods
	Abdomen tends to hang out
	Surface of abdomen is uneven and distended
	Use over-the-counter pain medications
_____ TOTAL	

0-4	ENERGY LEVELS
	Weakness
	Easily fatigued, sleepy during the day
	Fatigue is persistent and extreme
	Apathetic and lethargic
	Tired, even after a good night's rest
_____ TOTAL	

0-4	KIDNEY
	Urine has a strong odor
	Pain in mid-back region
	Urine is frothy
	Urinate infrequently
_____ TOTAL	

0-4	IMMUNE SYSTEM	0-4	OTHER
	Frequent infections (bladder, skin, ear, chest, sinus)		Food allergies
	Frequent colds or flu		Feel worse in moldy or musty places
_TOTAL		_TOTAL	

Please add the numbers from each section and write the total in the spaces provided, then add all the totals for each section together and put that total in the space below.

GRAND TOTAL: _____

How to interpret your score:
- **Less than or equal to 15:** Excellent
- **16-30:** Good
- **31-40:** Marginal
- **Greater than or equal to 51:** Very Poor

INDEX

DR. DANIEL KALISH

Daniel Kalish, D.C., is a pioneer, having developed his own clinical model of functional medicine which he now teaches to health care practitioners. The Kalish Method training seminar, a mentorship program in functional medicine, is a webinar-based training program founded on over eighteen years of clinical results from working with thousands of patients. Dr. Kalish teaches a logical sequence of therapeutic programs using the best lab tests available and focuses on how to communicate effectively with patients to correct chronic health conditions, and, importantly, how to build a thriving practice.

Dr. Kalish was recently invited to participate in the One Mind For Research group by the Honorable Patrick Kennedy. The first One Mind For Research conference in Boston in 2011 was a gathering of the top 200 neuroscientists in the United States, coming together to form a unified front to promote research on brain disorders.

For ten years Dr. Kalish directed The Natural Path Clinic in Del Mar, California, where he coordinated a team of medical doctors, nutritionists, chiropractors, and acupuncturists. Dr. Kalish now maintains an active international phone consultation practice.

In his private practice, Dr. Kalish has developed nutritional programs for a varied group of patients, over 8,000 in all, ranging from Olympic athletes to new moms. His programs are highly effective across a broad population with a variety of health complaints.

Dr. Kalish received his B.A. in Physiological Psychology from Antioch College, Yellow Springs, Ohio. He studied at the University of London and conducted research with biochemist Dr. Robin Monroe at Cambridge University. He also worked with renowned psychiatrist Dr. R.D. Lang utilizing drug-free treatments for schizophrenics.

Dr. Kalish spent two years in monastic training in Asia. He lived at a Zen monastery in Japan, where he studied organic farming, Zen meditation, and the art of Zen archery under Harada Roshi. He also lived in a forest monastery in Thailand studying meditation and the transcription of Buddhist texts for Vipassana master Achan Buddadasa. He is a certified Alexander Technique teacher and trained for two years with Marion Rosen, founder of Rosen Method Bodywork.

"I wrote this book both for health care practitioners and the public. A great interest in natural health solutions currently exists for those who have become somewhat disillusioned with the conventional medical approach to solving many common health problems. Unfortunately, I frequently get emails and calls from people searching in vain for health care practitioners experienced in this type of work, and vast areas of this country remain underserved. I see great demand from consumers to have easy access to these natural programs, but a lack of doctors to provide them. My hope is that this book will give you, the consumer, enough information to know what to look for in a natural health program, and that more practitioners will be encouraged to join the wave to make functional medicine an important part of their practice."

Daniel Kalish